T3-BPL-645

Effie Hanchett

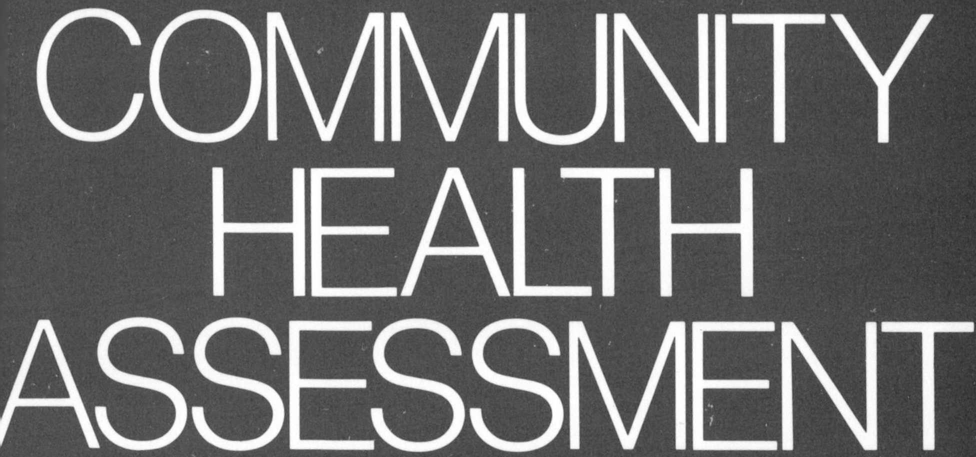

COMMUNITY HEALTH ASSESSMENT

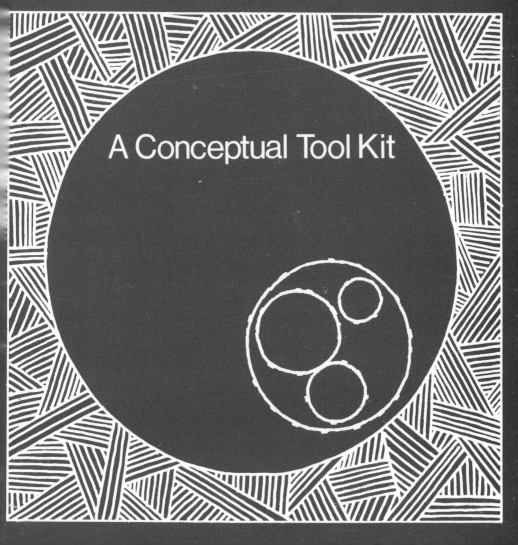

A Conceptual Tool Kit

Community Health Assessment: A Conceptual Tool Kit

COMMUNITY HEALTH ASSESSMENT:

A CONCEPTUAL TOOL KIT

Effie S. Hanchett, Ph.D., R.N.

Associate Professor
Faculty of Nursing
University of Toronto

Formerly, Program Director
Graduate Program in Community Health Nursing
School of Education, Health, Nursing,
and Arts Professions
Division of Nursing
New York University

A Wiley Medical Publication
JOHN WILEY & SONS
New York · Chichester · Brisbane · Toronto

Library of Congress Cataloging in Publication Data:

Hanchett, Effie S

Community health assessment.

(A Wiley medical publication)

Bibliography: p.

Includes index.

1. Community health nursing. 2. Public health—Evaluation. 3. System analysis. I. Title.

RT98.H36 610.73'43 78-13648

ISBN 0-471-34776-0

Printed in the United States of America

10 9 8 7 6 5 4 3 2 1

FOREWORD

In this book Dr. Hanchett has succeeded in presenting an innovative and humanistic learning tool for students of community health. Within this tool kit the reader will find a way of conceptualizing the complexities of community dynamics that is both adequate for a thorough assessment of a community's health (regardless of the size of the community under consideration) and facile enough to permit a creative approach to that assessment.

Basic to Dr. Hanchett's approach to community is the clear recognition that the community is made up of living people and that any assessment must be framed within the context of the human condition. Because the community is in constant, vital flux, to understand the principles that underlie this perpetually shifting milieu, one must be willing to recognize that the life forces involved in holding a community together are of a considerable depth and extend in many directions. There are no simplistic answers that are acceptable in an honest appraisal of communith health. Human beings are highly sophisticated living systems. The connecting activities that bind these individuals living in community are multifaceted and, therefore, a valid assessment must be devised that will encompass these several dimensions.

To provide a ledger for a multidimensional frame of reference, the outstanding characteristic of which is constant change, Dr. Hanchett has turned to computer science and chosen a humanized version of systems theory. This she has coupled with conceptualizations that derive from the perspective of new-age physics, in which physical conditions are no longer regarded as static; instead they are recognized as no more than the momentary nexus, or meeting place, of many—perhaps infinite—natural forces in a space-time, multidimensional universe.

Dr. Hanchett draws an analogue between the new-age scientist's analysis of the physical universe and the new-age community health nurse's assessment of the living human universe of community. Using a general systems approach, she demonstrates in her book that several concepts heretofore restricted to theory about the physical domain have relevance to the interrelationships of people in community. It is a daring leap to take but, once taken, it will open new vistas to community health assessment.

Dolores Krieger, Ph.D., R.N.
Professor of Nursing
New York University

PREFACE

Communities, the focus of community health nursing, constitute one of the major environmental forces in human health. Community provides the human element in man's environment and mediates other human and nonhuman factors. These run the gamut from material resources, such as nutritional elements and the patterning of their use by the human factor of culture, to human interactions and patterns of relationship with a larger force, be it that defined by science or by religion.

The individual's health is reflected in his community through his contributions to its statistical rates as well as to the cultural and emotional tone of the community. Conversely, the community is reflected in the individual through the same variety of expressions.

The purpose of this *Tool Kit* is to set down a beginning framework and principles of community health along with some suggested resources so that individual students and nurses working in community health can use and evolve these principles to their own use and to the benefit of the communities they serve.

This book began as a series of "droodles" to illustrate basic principles to be applied to community during the time I was teaching graduate students in community health nursing at New York University. It continued to evolve in response to the need and interest expressed by a variety of people for a basic resource for teaching community health nursing at all educational levels.

Much of the *Tool Kit* is the result of mulling over ideas gleaned from a great variety of sources—books, conversations, struggles to be. Where it is possible to document a source so that the reader might pursue it, it is footnoted. If I have unwittingly incorporated something into my own philosophy so completely that I am no longer aware of the source, I apologize.

This *Tool Kit* is dedicated to the many people who contributed greatly to its accomplishment, although the responsibility for any of its flaws is certainly my own. It is impossible to identify all the contributors by name. However, special mention is due to some. Those who preceded me at New York University and who contributed to the development of that program and consequently to this *Tool Kit* include Jeannette Spero and Gail Malloy, Kate Ahmadi, and Carmen

McLean. Joyce Fitzpatrick and Henrietta Blackman, who worked with me, and Mary Jane Pirie, who succeeded me, also contributed by sharing their insights and views. Special credit is due to the students whose use and questioning of principles provided additional insights, and to Martha Rogers, Chairman of the Department of Nursing Education at N.Y.U., who created and maintained an atmosphere in which intellectual curiosity, commitment, and enthusiasm were encouraged.

I am also grateful to those who helped make the production of this book possible. Lena Butterfield, who typed the manuscript, Guy Smalley, who redrew the illustrations, Kenny Beck for the design, and Eileen Tommaso who supervised the various stages of production.

Particular credit is due to Joanne Griffin, whose recognition of and enthusiasm for the *Tool Kit* were largely responsible for its continuing development, and to my editors at Wiley, Earl Shepherd and Cathy Somer, who were both willing to risk and who kept me plodding along in spite of my own tight schedules in other areas. Credit, too, is due to Robert Logan of the Department of Physics at the University of Toronto, who provided a last check on some of the principles from physics.

Finally, an immense debt of gratitude is owed to Florence Downs, whose amazing ability to perceive the value of an idea, while maintaining the ability to perceive and to ask the difficult questions to hone and clarify that idea, has contributed greatly to this effort.

This *Tool Kit* is also dedicated to you, its readers, who, it is my hope, will take these principles, test them, refine them, and hopefully assist communities in developing as dynamic, constructive environments for human health.

Effie S. Hanchett, Ph.D., R.N.

CONTENTS

Community Health Assessment: A Conceptual Tool Kit

Introduction

Background and Rationale

The concept of community as the focus for nursing assessment and intervention has roots both old and new to public health nursing. Lillian Wald took social and political action to change the conditions on the Lower East Side of New York during the early part of this century (Wald, 1915). Jeannette Spero made the concept of community the focus of nursing assessment and intervention in nursing education during the early 1960's through her innovative revision of the Master's Program in Public Health Nursing at New York University (Spero, 1977).

Every professional nurse, as she comes to know her individual patients in increasing depth, begins to recognize the forces within the family which affect the health of that individual. For example, family forces which affect the health of the individual are seen in the effect of a mother's depleted emotional or economic resources on the health of her child. Every nurse who follows a family in depth begins to recognize forces within the community which affect the health of families. Some community forces which affect the health of families are seen in 1) high unemployment rates and consequent poverty, and 2) inadequate access to medical care due to economic, transportation, or other barriers.

Community forces do affect the health of individuals and of families. Direct assessment of and intervention with the community and its forces constitutes a complex challenge to nursing activity. Through assessment, the health of many individuals may be indirectly affected without continuous direct delivery of nursing interventions to every community member.

The Tools

The tools for assessment of the community are provided by general systems approaches. One aspect of a general systems approach focuses on identifying a system, its subsystems, and suprasystem and the relationships between these. This approach can serve as a powerful tool to cut through the complexities and identify the many interacting relationships within a complex system such as a community. The general systems approach to identifying a system and its relationships is presented in Part 1 of this *Tool Kit* (Chapter 1).

The concept of health implies energy, individuality, relationships, and continuing progress toward developmental tasks. A wide variety of concepts drawn from many diverse disciplines, such as physics, psychology, and from communication and developmental theories, can contribute to an understanding of health. Basic elements in a concept of health are presented in Part 2 of this *Tool Kit* (Chapters 2 through 8).

The tools for assessment of the level of health of any given system can be drawn from many sources. Another aspect of a general systems approach focuses on the applicability of basic principles across many different disciplines. Principles which are true for one living system will hold true for another living system (Bertalanffy, 1955). Consequently, concepts for assessment of the level of health have been drawn from a variety of sources—communication and developmental theories, principles of goal-directed behaviors, and principles from physics. These principles provide the discrete tools to facilitate assessment of the level of wellness of the system under consideration. Basic concepts relevant to health are presented under "Health" at the beginning of each unit in Part 2 of this *Tool Kit*.

The concept of community health requires the integration of concepts and values regarding the community and concepts related to health. One aspect of a general systems approach provides a framework by which to identify a specific community, its parts, and their relationships. Another approach provides relevant concepts from a variety of sources to facilitate identification of the sources of wellness and barriers to continuing development in any given community. Examples of applications of a concept of health within a particular community situation are presented under "Community Health," the second element within each unit in Part 2.

Questions and suggestions related to the concept of health with possible relevance for the community selected for study are presented under "Community Health Assessment," the third element of each unit in Part 2.

Many concepts gleaned from a variety of sources are presented for use in identifying and assessing the sources of, and barriers to, wellness within a community. The power of the concepts results from their interaction with each other, and their application by a real person in a real setting—Just as is the case with other community assessment tools of a map, census tract statistics, and a person to read these, observe the community, and identify the relationship between the quality of life observed, the location, and the statistical information. The person who uses the tools must choose the tools which are most appropriate to the specific setting and task at hand.

The community which you assess, the specific concepts which you choose to pursue in that community, and the interactions between you—the assessor—the community, and the concepts can provide a powerful force with which to assist a community in identifying and planning for its own priorities in increasing its wellness and, consequently, the health of the individuals and families for whom it is home.

Organization of this Tool Kit

This book is organized into two main parts. The first part deals with the tools of general systems theory. It introduces the concepts of system, subsystem, suprasystem, and relationships. These are necessary to define a specific community for your assessment of its level of wellness.

The second part of the book simply provides a number of concepts, or tools, which can be used to identify and describe the forces affecting the health of a given community. These concepts will be more useful to you if you have a specific community in mind. It is up to you to read with a critical eye, and identify which of the concepts presented have relevance—that is, which will work—for you in describing the forces for wellness in the community which you have selected for study.

Each concept is presented in the form of a figure. For those of you who are visual thinkers, this will serve as the primary source for the concept. Written clarification of each of the concepts is presented on the two pages associated with each figure. The written clarification is organized according to three headings. The first heading, "Health," presents the basic concept with its implications for the health of any living system. These implications may be stated explicitly or implied by virtue of their content.

The second heading, "Community Health," provides examples of the concept applied to situations within community.

The third heading, "Community Health Assessment," presents examples of questions which result from considering the concept of health in relation to community. These are presented primarily for their value in clarifying the use of the concept. They are *not* intended as a specific guide to the assessment of any community's level of health. The relevant questions for assessment of any specific community's health can, at this time, be identified only from the questions raised by listening to and observing the community itself.*

References

Bertalanffy, Ludwig von. General system theory. *Main Currents in Modern Thought*, 1955, *11*, 75–83.

Spero, Jeannette R. *New trends in the educational preparation of community health nurse specialists*. Conference of Community Health Nursing Educa-

*I first became acquainted with the use of "community," "health," "community health," "assessment," and "community health assessment" as organizing concepts for teaching public health nursing in 1970 through Ms. Kate Ahmadi.

tion and Service Representatives, Simmons College, Boston, Mass., April 1969.

Spero, Jeannette R. An Overview of Health—Health A Community Systems Model. National League for Nursing. Publication: Maintaining Health—An Adventure in Transition, 1973.

Wald, Lillian. *The House on Henry Street*. New York: Holt, Rinehart & Winston, 1915. (Reprinted, New York: Dover, 1971.)

1

PART ONE

Defining and Describing a Community Using General Systems Theory

Concepts from general systems theory are presented for use in defining and describing a community as the focus of nursing assessment.

1

CHAPTER ONE

General Systems Theory and the Community

General systems theory intends to cut through professional jargon by identifying principles common to many disciplines. Community—people in relationship with others—can serve as a system that can be defined and described, both as a whole and in terms of its parts and their relationships.

General Systems Theory

The basic notion of general systems theory is that knowledge can be broken down into basic principles that will work—that is, they will hold true—for everything that falls within the unit (system) identified (Bertalanffy, 1955, pp. 75–77).

General systems theorists seek to reduce the negative impact of professional jargon that keeps bits of knowledge useful to only one field. Professional jargon keeps people with information about one thing separated from people with information about another thing. The general systems approach attempts to increase the dialogue between people by giving them a common language.

It is exciting to search for basic principles in a language which can be understood by all. The potential gain for all fields of endeavor is immense. The distribution of resources provides an example of a concept common to many fields of inquiry. Principles describing the means by which the distribution of resources occurs can be identified by many fields of inquiry—physics, information theory, sociology, and economics to name a few. Many of the principles identified will work for other fields of study. When they do not, it is because of intervening variables that may or may not be unique to the system in question. The identification of these intervening variables and their impact further enriches the understanding of the original principle. The clarification that results, in turn, enriches the information available to workers in all fields.

The vocabulary of general systems theory is intended to be clear, concise, and equally understandable to all. However, somehow in the process of its development the term "systems" has become associated with computer systems and computer technology and general systems approaches have become confused with computer systems approaches. Much of the language of both general and computer systems theories has become incorporated. Planners and those who use computers find systems and organization theory valuable in dealing with large numbers of people. The language of computers does not communicate well unique human experience and values. It is geared toward identifying the countable, measurable descriptors of things. As a result, the language of systems theory often sounds dehumanized.

The principles of general systems theory, especially when expressed in nonjargonistic terms, can contribute a great deal to the understanding of people by people.

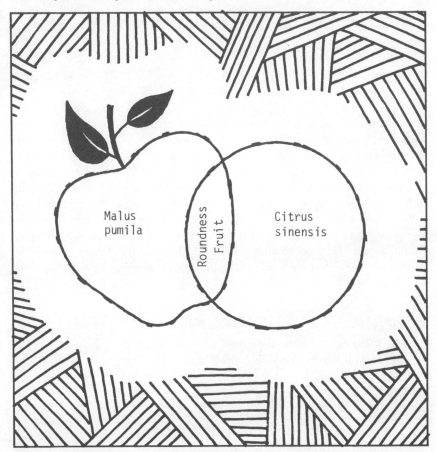

The Latin name for apple is *Malus pumila*. The proper botanist's name for an orange is *Citrus sinensis*. Both are fruit, both are round. Many more people (consumers, nutritionists, agriculturalists, community organizers, and supermarket managers, for example) can talk intelligently about apples and oranges, roundness, and fruit than can talk about *Malus pumila* and *Citrus sinensis* (Stern, 1966).

Community as System

HUMAN SYSTEMS

Nurses and nursing deal with human "systems." There are many "sizes" of human "systems" that a nurse may choose for her area of focus.

The individual is the basic unit of any of these. Some nurses choose to focus on individuals as the unit for assessment and intervention. As one becomes more and more aware of the forces affecting the health of individuals, it becomes increasingly evident that the family, and the health and dynamics of the family as a whole, have a tremendous impact on the health of individuals. Once again, as one becomes increasingly aware of the factors and forces which affect the health of families, one becomes increasingly aware of the impact of the community on the health of families. The economic health of the community affects the economic health of the family, and therefore its nutritional, physical and emotional health as well. The community's culture, values, and attitudes about child rearing practices affect the health of the individuals within the family and of the family as a whole.

DEFINITION OF A COMMUNITY AS SYSTEM

To focus on a community as a system requires an understanding of the concept of community. Most definitions of community include four basic elements:

1. People
2. Place
3. Resources and services
4. Relationships between the people, and between the people, the place, and the resources (Suttles, 1968; Stern, 1967; Warren, 1963)

People in relationship to one another are the essential elements of community. In most communities, place is one of the strongest elements holding people together. However, in other communities, a common goal, a common perspective, or a common need provide the "glue" of the relationship. Professional communities with their members scattered across the country have goals and interests as their common bond and no geographical boundaries (Warren, 1963). Communities of addicts have a need as their common bond. In most communities, varying needs, interests, and goals provide the relationship which binds people together. Whatever the reasons, communities of all types provide some sort of identity and "home base" to their people.

SELECTING A COMMUNITY FOR STUDY

Your reasons for deciding to do a community health assessment will affect your choice of community for study. If you are a member of a community

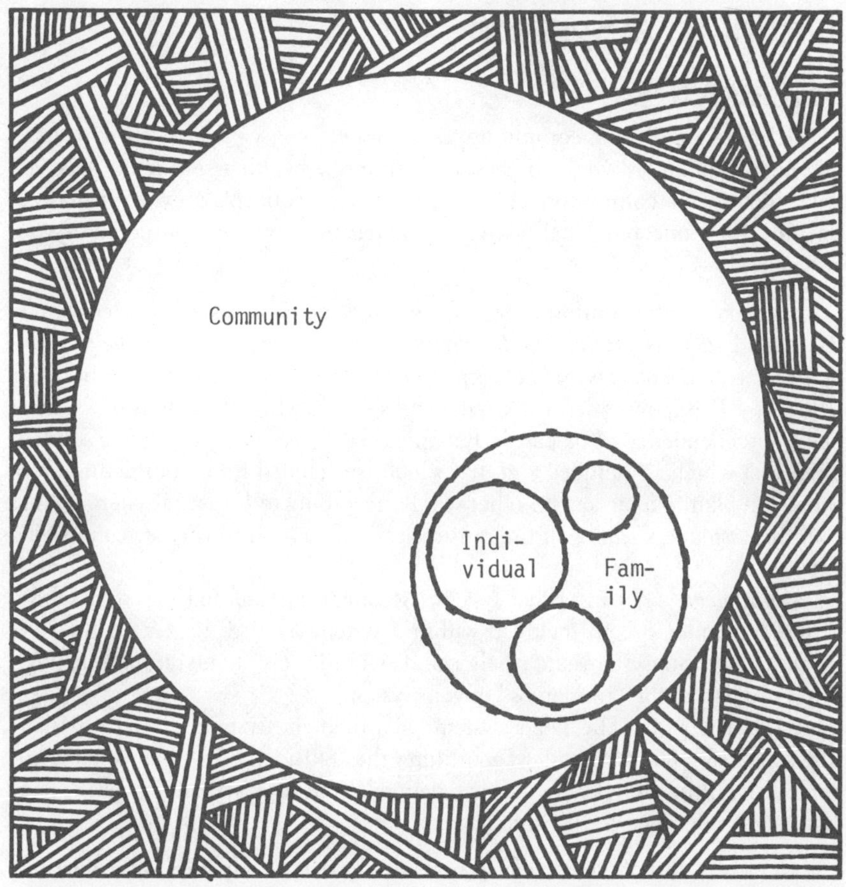

planning board, your community will be that of the defined area to which you are accountable. If you desire to study a community which supports the agency which employs you, your choice will be that community, or a part of the larger community which supports the services of your agency. If you are studying the health of a community in your role as student you have more choices open to you, but a less clear rationale to collect the information which you will need. In any case, your interests, your values and the interest and accessibility of a community provide the initial directions for selecting a community for study. A community where you live or work, or one which has asked for some assistance, provides the best starting point.

Defining a System

THE WORDS

Defining a specific community as the system you wish to focus on is often the most difficult task in the process of community health assessment. Once you have identified a community for study, three basic concepts provide the tools to identify the conceptual boundaries of that community for purposes of your assessment.

System. The community itself, no more, no less. A system, according to Hall and Fagen, *is a set of objects* (components, parts) *together with the relationships between the objects and between their attributes* (Hall & Fagen, in Buckley, 1968, p. 81). Rapoport defined a system as "a whole which functions by virtue of the interdependence of its parts" (Rapoport, 1968, p. xvii). A system also identifies that which is included and that which is excluded from your definition of what you plan to focus on. In other words, according to Fuller, a system defines "all the insideness" and "all the outsideness" of your, in this case, community (1969).

Subsystem. A part of that system. According to Hall and Fagen, a subsystem is a smaller system included within a system (Hall & Fagen, in Buckley, 1968, p. 84). Subsystems are smaller units within the system you have defined. They are part of the "insideness" of your system.

Suprasystem. The larger system, of which the system is a part (Miller, 1965, p. 218). The suprasystem constitutes the "outsideness"—that which is not included within the system you have defined. The suprasystem, however, does have great relevance to the system.

A critical part of the concept of system is the dynamic quality of the relationships between all aspects of the system and its environment. Relationships between subsystems, system and subsystems, and between system and suprasystem must be considered for a full understanding of the dynamics of any given system.

The nesting of relationships between system, subsystem and suprasystem was stated by Alan Watts using the notion of (energy) fields.

Little fields have big fields
Upon their backs to bite 'em,
And big fields have bigger fields,
And so, ad infinitum.

From Alan Watts, *On the Taboo Against Knowing Who You Are,* p. 89, copyright © 1966, Pantheon Books, a Division of Random House, Inc. Used by permission.

Hall and Fagen used a stereo system as an example of a system with its components, and the relationships between its components. The system—the stereo as a whole, and its subsystem (or components)—the receiver, the speakers, and the turntable—must all be connected if the system is to work (Hall & Fagen, in Buckley, 1968, pp. 83–84).

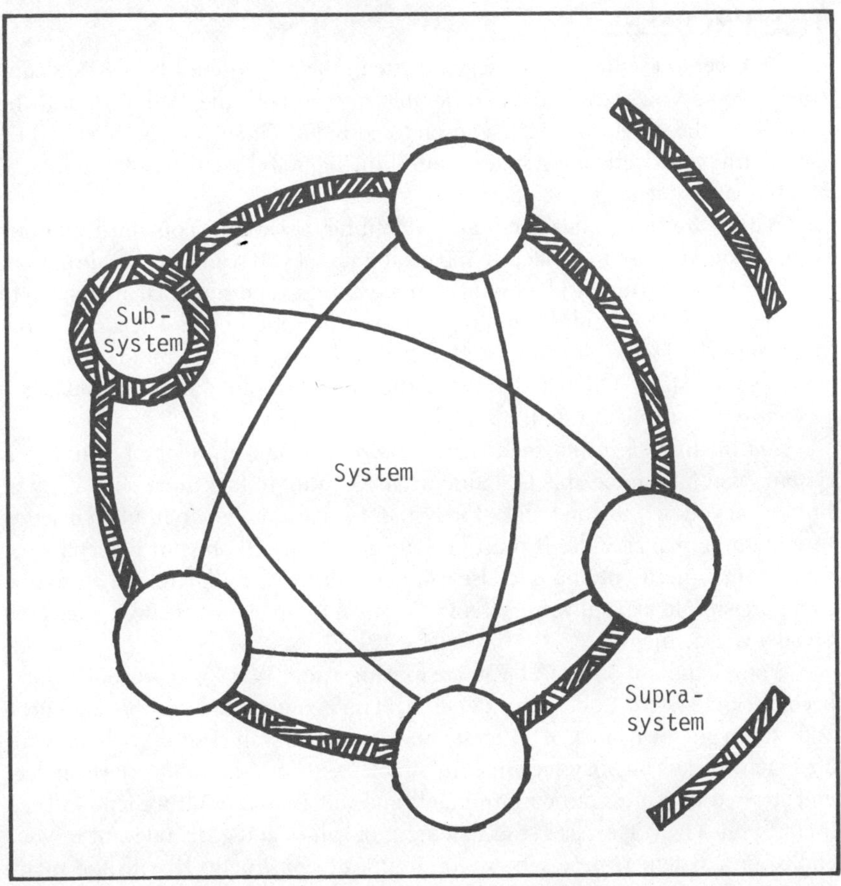

System: a set of objects (components, parts) together with the relationships between the objects and between their attributes (Hall & Fagen, in Buckley, 1968, p. 81).
Subsystem: a smaller system included within a system (Hall & Fagen, in Buckley, 1968, p. 84).
Suprasystem: a larger system which includes the system under consideration.

If the system is not working properly, that is, if you cannot get any music, it may be the result of a problem with one of the connections (or relationships) between the components, just as well as with one of the components themselves. For the system to function intact, functioning relationships between the parts are necessary.

Additional relationships with the environment are also necessary. The system must be connected to a source of electricity, the receiver must be able to pick up radio waves, or someone must place a record or tape in the proper position. A person is usually required to "flip the switch" and is certainly required to hear the music and value it sufficiently to do what is necessary to adjust and maintain the system.

THE PROCESS

In order to use the tools of general systems theory you must bc able to define your system. You must know and be able to state both the "WHAT" and the "WHY" of the system you have chosen to consider. Otherwise you may end up considering two overlapping systems but thinking that these two systems are one and the same system.

There are three considerations in defining a system. You must contract (focus in on) the system by identifying what it is that you really want to deal with. You must also expand by identifying as many things as possible that are related to what you want to consider. Finally, you must find the line that separates what you want to include within your system from what you do not want to consider as part of your system. This will define "all the insideness" and "all the outsideness" of your system (Fuller, 1969).

Contracting, focusing in on the problem, is one element of defining a system. You have to be able to define what you want to look at carefully. It will limit what you see, so don't make the system too narrow, but do limit your scope to something manageable. It must be *your* choice, based on your perception of some human need, and no one else can define it for you. (There will always be some pressure to expand your system to include more elements, no matter how broadly you define it.)

Your definition of WHAT you are looking at and WHY you are looking at it becomes the system under consideration. This requires that you both identify and state your own area of interest, and your own values and goals in your approach to it. You may feel uncomfortable. Our culture often make us feel embarrassed to express our commitments and values; as a result we tend to keep them to ourselves. However, the statement of values and goals relevant to your choice of a system is necessary to communicate constructively with the many other people who are involved with that system.

Suppose, for example, that you are interested in the local hospital's emergency room (the WHAT of your system). The hospital administrator is also looking at the hospital's emergency room (the same WHAT for his system).

However, you are looking at it from the point of view of a community advocate, knowing the community's need for a 24-hour walk-in clinic (your WHY). The hospital administrator is looking at it from the point of view of the hospital's need to curtail services, knowing the hospital's need to freeze staffing and curtail costs to avoid an impending financial disaster (the administrator's WHY). You are both talking about the same emergency room. You both think you are talking about the same thing. Well, you are, and then again, you aren't. If you can find out what is common and what is not common to your two viewpoints, then you will be able to proceed much more easily and much more rapidly (Bennis, Benne, & Chin, 1969). You can go on to identify further commonalities or to realize that you cannot, but you can do so in such a way that you can maintain your relationship and return to talk to each other for other purposes at another time.

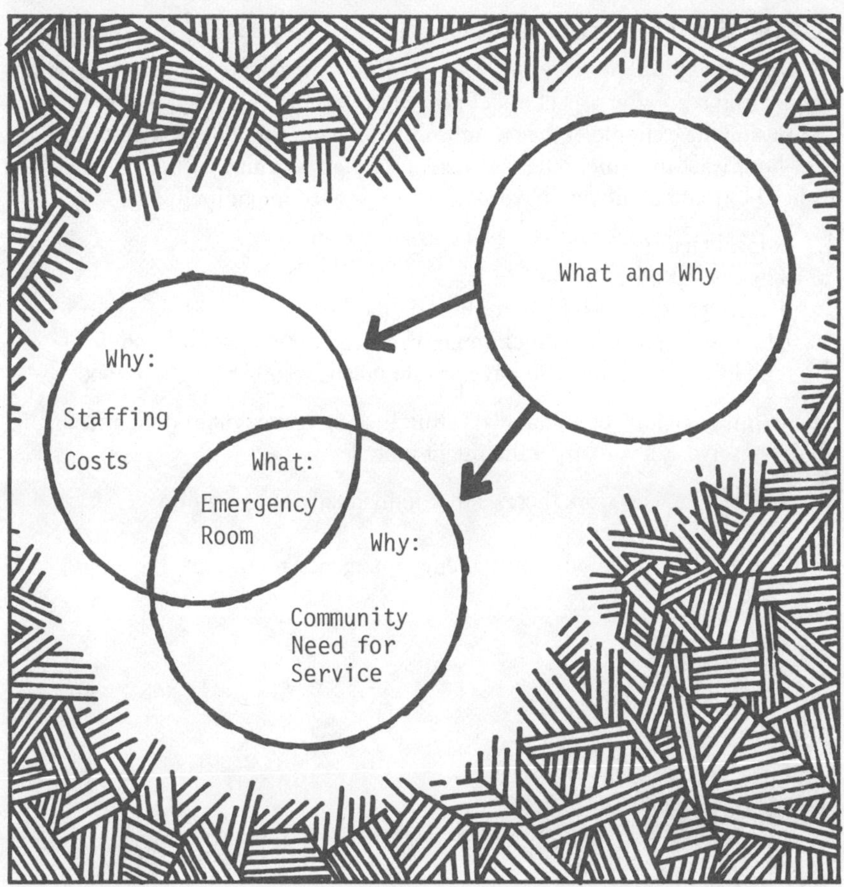

In order to define a system, you need both your system (the WHAT) as an area of investigation and your reason (the WHY), your value-based goals, for considering it.

Know and be able to state your system (WHAT and WHY), and if you are negotiating with someone, be able to get that person to identify his. The lack of clarity about different goals (WHY) in discussing the same thing (WHAT) is often the point of discrepancy where misunderstanding begins.

You cannot understand or deal with the administrator's overall budget requirements. That is not your system, nor can the administrator deal with the totality of your system. Both of your values, goals, and loyalties are rightfully rooted in different and acceptable reference groups.

IDENTIFY THE ELEMENTS

Identifying all the elements that have an impact on the system you are considering is another aspect of defining your system.

Using the example of the community from your point of view of its need for a 24-hour walk-in clinic, other subsystems of the community which might affect its need for, and ability to deliver, a 24-hour service might include:

1. A local factory
2. The nearest other hospital
3. The older people who live in the neighborhood
4. The working people with children who live in the neighborhood
5. The local physicians who have private practices in the neighborhood

These things (factors, components) within the emergency room itself affecting its ability to serve as a walk-in clinic might include:

1. The people who work there, either individually or as a group
2. The available space
3. The available methods for financing emergency room visits

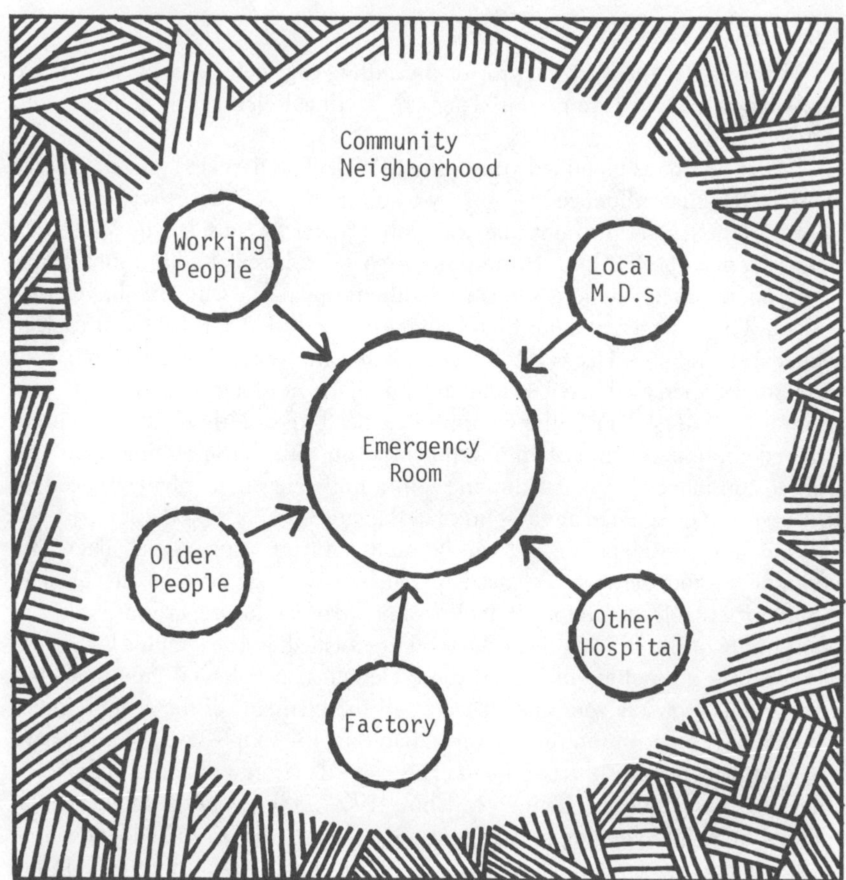

After you have identified the WHAT and WHY of your system, you need to identify those things which have an impact on your system. Think of all the possible things which could affect the system you are considering—whether from inside the system itself or from its environment.

DRAW THE LINE

Drawing the line that will provide the cutting edge between what is included and what is excluded from your system, is a critical element in defining your system.

After you have identified your system (WHAT and WHY) and considered those factors that influence it, you may well find that it is necessary to redefine your system. It may turn out that you would prefer to consider the WHAT of your system to be the local community itself. The hospital administrator may well decide that he or she has to consider the hospital as a whole as the relevant system. The emergency room then becomes the relevant subsystem for each of your considerations. His WHY for considering the system includes both your requests for increased services and the hospital's need for keeping costs to a minimum. Your WHY is the community's need for a 24-hour walk-in clinic. The redefinition of your system now provides you with a clear cutting edge. You want to consider everything within the community relevant to solving its need for the service. The services and resources of the larger city of which it is a part will also demand consideration, but will be excluded from your system. There is a constant tension between the need to redefine your system and the need to maintain a stable definition of that system in order to properly assess it. In community health, that cutting edge is often provided by a geographic boundary. The pressure to include more and more elements, people and groups, within your system grows as your knowledge of all the elements of the system grows. There is only one common-sense way of handling it—simply say, "This is what I can cope with. This is the bite I can chew, and therefore I'm going to draw the line right here (Bennis, Benne, & Chin, 1969). I'll recognize other factors, identify them as belonging to the suprasystem, but I will not include the whole world in my assessment." For example, if the local community of 250,000 people in which the emergency room exists is our system, the city of 2 million people of which the local community is a part then becomes its suprasystem. The emergency room is then defined as a subsystem of the local community.

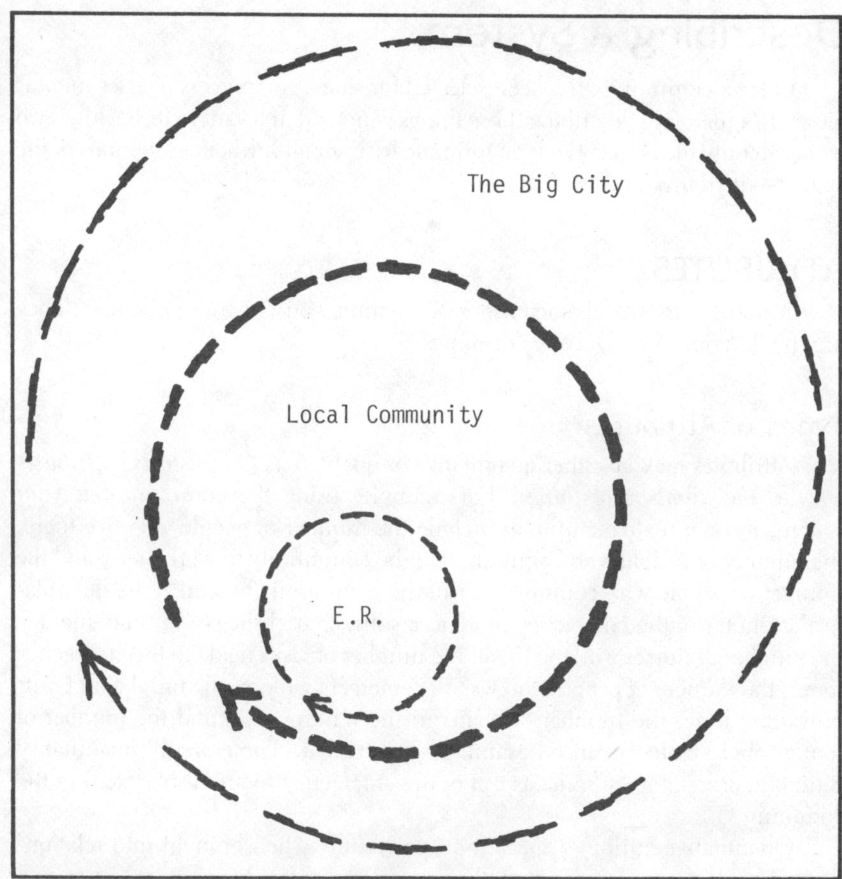

After considering all those things which may affect your system, *draw the line*. Make a decision about what you will include and what you will exclude from your system.

Describing a System

Once a community has been selected for study, the process of assessment is basically a matter of describing those things which are relevant to its health. Two words identify the concepts which form the basis for all further descriptions of the system—*attributes* and *relationships*.

ATTRIBUTES

Attributes are the characteristics of anything you choose to describe. They are the descriptors of processes or things.

Types of Attributes

Attributes may be either quantitative or qualitative. *Quantitative attributes refer to the numbers of things.* For example, using the community as your system, its quantitative attributes include the number of people who live there, the number of people who commute into the community to work there, and the number of people who commute out of the community to work. The quantitative attributes of the emergency room as a subsystem of the community include the number of nurses working there, the number of visits made to the emergency room, the number of people who visit the emergency room, the number of hours of waiting time, the number of chairs in the waiting area, and the number of rooms where patients can be examined and treated. These are all quantitative (number) descriptors of some aspect of the emergency room (a subsystem of the community).

Quantitative attributes speak most powerfully when brought into relationship. The 100 people who visit the emergency room between 8:00 P.M. and midnight wait an average of one and a half hours to be seen while the 25 people who visit the emergency room between midnight and 8:00 A.M. wait an average of 30 minutes to be seen.

Qualitative attributes refer to the character, nature or distinguishing aspect of a thing. Qualitative attributes of the community as a system include the people's perception of their own health, medical care in general, and of the quality of care provided by the emergency room in particular. Qualitative attributes of the emergency room as a subsystem include the quality of the waiting room—bright and cheerful, or dingy; the quality of the care given—excellent, adequate, or inadequate; and the quality of relationships with the emergency room clients—warm, caring, unhurried or cold, unfeeling, and rushed. Relationships can exist between different quantitative attributes and between quantitative and qualitative attributes. For example, 85 percent of the people who visit the emergency room feel that they get adequate care. Some 25 percent of the people who visit the emergency room feel that the care provided is caring and unrushed.

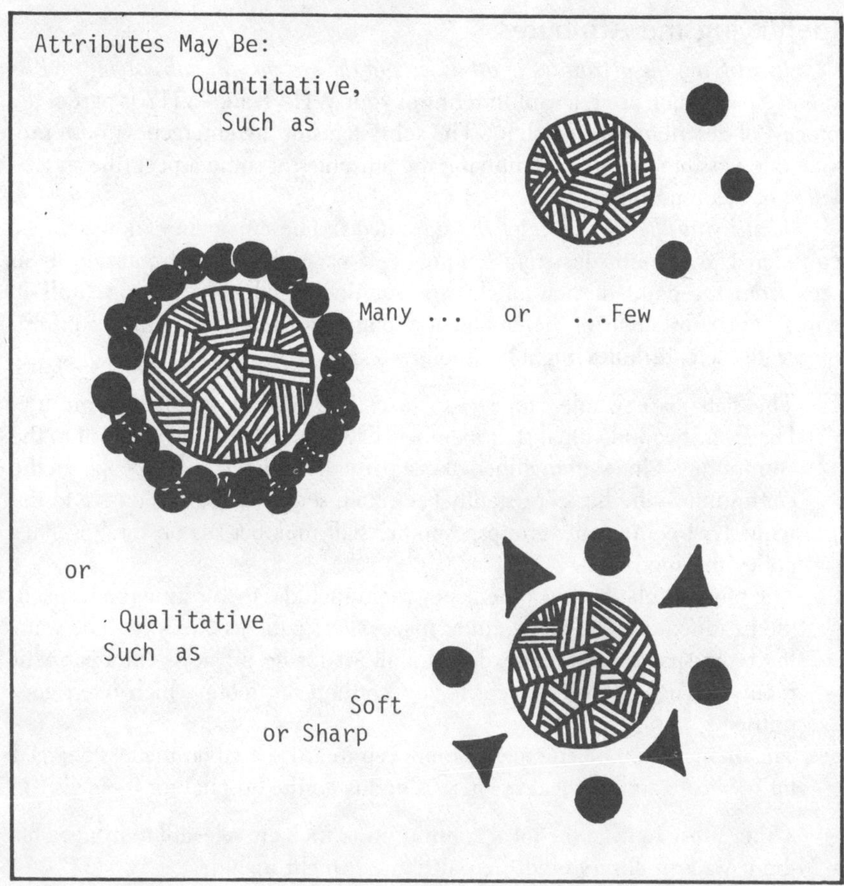
Attributes May Be:
Quantitative,
Such as
Many ... or ...Few
or
Qualitative
Such as
Soft
or Sharp

Attributes are the characteristics of anything you choose to describe. Attributes may be quantitative; that is, they may describe whatever it is in terms of numbers, or they may be qualitative, and describe it in terms of kind.

Identifying the Attributes

Identifying the attributes of all aspects of the system, the subsystem, and its suprasystem which are relevant in terms of your WHAT and WHY is part of the process of describing your system. The subsystems of the emergency room provide one possible focus for identifying the attributes of some aspect (the subsystems) of a community.

Identifying the attributes of the subsystems. The emergency room may be considered to be one subsystem (component, part) of the local community as seen from the point of view of the community's need for a 24-hour walk-in clinic. The subsystems of the emergency room (sub-subsystems of the community) with their attributes might be as follows:

1. The staff, as a whole, appears to take little interest in the community. However, two individual staff members have special interests relevant to the community. One staff member takes a particular interest in the people in the community. She has consistently been both sensitive and responsive to the requests of community groups. Another staff member sits on the hospital's policy-making board.
2. The physical plant of the emergency room includes the waiting room space, the treatment rooms, and counter space where patients check in. The waiting room space is often crowded and allows for no privacy. The treatment rooms are usually full, except for one orthopedic room which often goes unused.
3. The financing of the emergency room is primarily based on the fees charged for medicare and medicaid. There is no loss to the hospital for these visits.

Other subsystems of the local community (which are relevant to its need for a 24-hour walk-in clinic), and their attributes, might include:

1. The local factory, which runs on a 24-hour-a-day schedule and has its own physician on call. The management of the factory is concerned about a potential increase in its real estate tax. As a result, it has considered relocating to the suburbs.
2. The nearest other hospital, a municipal hospital. Its emergency room is overwhelmed and people often wait for three or four hours before they can be seen by a physician.
3. Five private physicians, who serve the area. One of them is planning to retire and move out of the community during the next year. He is interested in, and active in the community.
4. A large number of working people with children, who live in a middle-income high rise building. They often wait for a husband or wife to return home from work before going to the emergency room in order that they needn't take all the children along with them.
5. Many older people, who live in buildings scattered throughout the area. They spend much of their time during the day sitting on park benches. They are afraid to go out of their apartments at night.

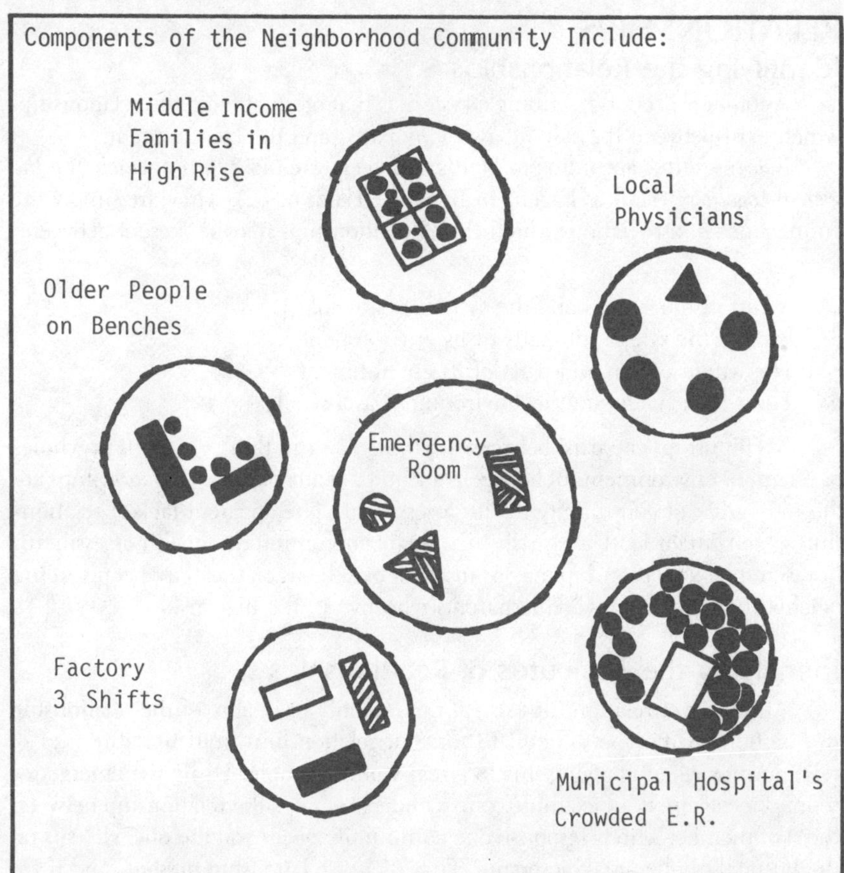

The tasks involved in describing a system include identifying the attributes of all relevant subsystems and elements of the suprasystem.

Attributes related to the entire city as the suprasystem include:

1. The city government, which is concerned about keeping jobs in the area in order to maintain its income from taxes.
2. The city department of hospitals, which is interested in reducing or limiting the number of visits to its own municipal hospital's emergency room.
3. The city department of social services, which is under tremendous pressure to cut down on the number of people receiving support due to unemployment.

RELATIONSHIPS

Identifying the Relationships

Another aspect of describing a system is that of identifying the relationships which exist between the system, its many parts, and the environment.

Relationships, according to Hall and Fagen, *are those things which "tie the system together*" (Hall & Fagen, in Buckley, 1968, p. 82). They are simply the connections or associations which exist. Relationships may be present between:

1. Parts of the system
2. A part of the system and the system as a whole
3. Parts of the sytem and parts of its environment
4. The whole system and parts of its environment
5. The whole system and its environment as a whole

Relationships can exist between anything you can think of—parts or wholes of system or environment, or between attributes of any of these. Relationships are the nitty-gritty of community health assessment. The apparent lack of relationship which might exist is equally significant in community health assessment. For example, a relationship may or may not exist between the older people in the neighborhood and the working parents who live in the high rise.

Identifying the Attributes of Relationships

Attributes of relationships reveal the quantity or quality of the relationship in question. It may be difficult to sort out relationships from the attributes of relationships when applying this to a real-world example. Using the emergency room once again as an example, one wonders "what is the relationship between the staff member who is responsive to community needs and the one who sits on the hospital's policy-making board? That is, is a relationship present, and if so, what is the quality of it? Do they talk to and respect each other? Does no relationship mean a negative relationship, or just the lack of time or opportunity to build a relationship? What kind of communication occurs between them? Can the person who sits on the Board hear messages about the community's needs and respect or support them?"

Questions about the relationships between the groups within the community might include:

"Do the residents of the middle-income high rise building know and trust any of the older residents well enough to allow them to baby sit? Is there a positive relationship? Do the older people fear those who live in the high rise? Is the relationship negative? Is there any contact between the local factory and the municipal hospital? Could the local factory get a tax rebate for using its on-call physician to assist in the emergency room at night and thereby free personnel to cover for a walk-in clinic?" This would relieve some of the load from walk-in clients at the municipal hospital.

"Could the private physician who is planning to leave town be persuaded to stay and help out in the emergency room on a part-time basis?"

Would it be possible to arrange for the older people to baby sit so mothers

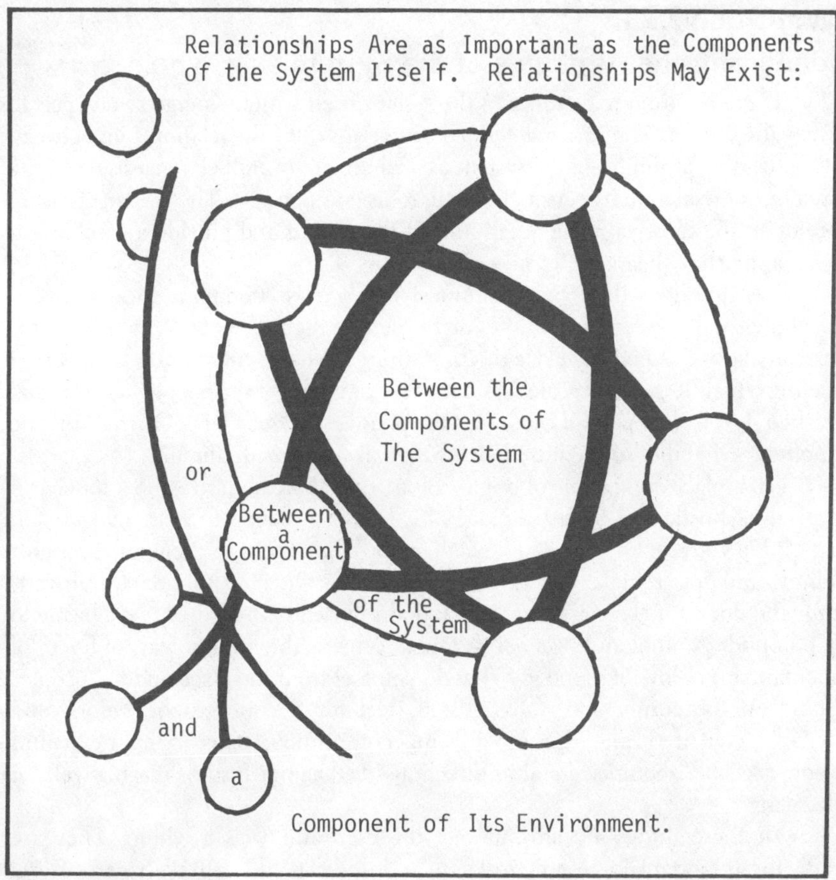
Relationships Are as Important as the Components
of the System Itself. Relationships May Exist:
Between the
Components of
The System
or
Between
a
Component
of the
System
and
a
Component of Its Environment.

Tasks involved in describing a system include:
Identifying the existing and potential relationships between:

1. The components or parts of the system
2. The parts of the system and the system as a whole
3. The parts of the system and parts of its environment
4. The system as a whole and parts of its environment
5. The system as a whole and its environment as a whole

Describing the attributes of the relationships:

1. Quantitative attributes
2. Qualitative attributes

could take their children to the clinic during the day rather than in the evening? This would ease demand for late night services and also provide income for the older people.

Would it be possible to set up a day care center in the local factory for working parents? They could leave their children there when they went to the clinic. Could the center be staffed by older people? Would the city be willing to provide tax relief for this?

WHOLENESS

Identifying the Attributes of the System as a Whole

There are unique qualities of the system itself which emerge as one gets to know the system. They are not defined by its parts or by the relationships between its parts. The attributes of the system as a whole are overall characteristics of the system, more akin to its personality than to its components. These characteristics are often the most valuable descriptors of the system and provide a baseline for evaluating the "meaning" of other descriptors.

The questions that come to mind when one is attempting to identify the attributes of the system as a whole might include the following: What is it that is special about this person, place or community? What is the unique character or feeling which it communicates? What issues or goals get the people to act? What is their level of hope? Of vitality? Of openness to outsiders? Of trust in one another? Of ability to identify their own goals and pursue them?

Is it a place and people of bright colors, or is there a more somber tone? Is it a place of hustle and bustle, a place of calm, or a place which is strangely too quiet? Do you feel energized or devitalized by being there? Is the weather bright, sunny, and does it make you want to be outdoors? Or is it damp, dark, introverting, and does it make you want to be indoors curled up by a fire? Is it a hassle to get around? A problem to get across town? What is the level of fear, of hope, of spontaneity, of joy, of sadness? What do you feel from the place and the people? Stand on the corner and watch, listen, feel for the movement, colors, and "vibes." Is it a young, vibrant, growing community, or is it mature, calm, knowledgeable about itself and its directions? Is it aging? If so, is it aging well, or decaying?

All these things are attributes of the community as a whole. They are critically important in coming to know and understand its strengths, resources, and needs for improvement.

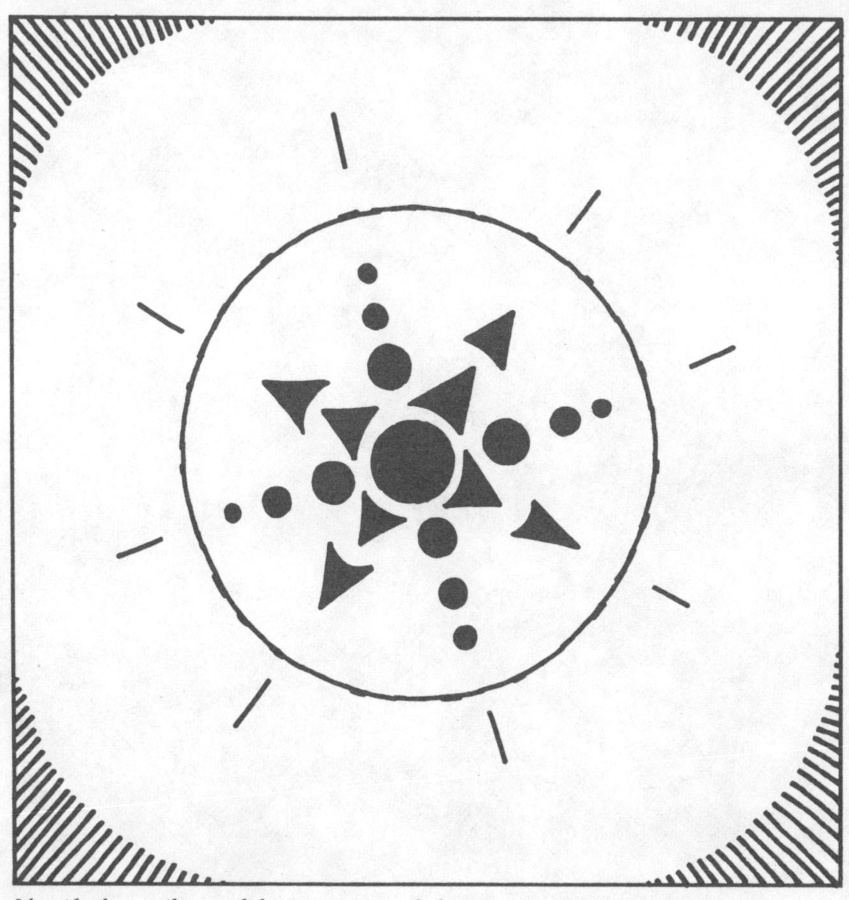

Identify the attributes of the system as a whole.

Any system you are considering has its own unique qualities or characteristics which are different from those of its parts.

"The whole is greater than the sum of its parts." (Miller, Living systems: basic concepts, 1965, p. 217; Rogers, 1970, p. 47).

The personality of a human being, the character of a neighborhood, a village, a city, or a town needs to be perceived or else what makes it unique or special will be lost.

References and Resources

REFERENCES

Bennis, Warren, Benne, Kenneth, & Chin, Robert (eds.). *The Planning of Change.* New York: Holt, Rinehart & Winston, 1969.

Bertalanffy, Ludwig von. General system theory. *Main Currents in Modern Thought*, 1955, 2, 75–83.

Buckley, Walter (ed.). *Modern Systems Research for the Behavioral Scientist: A Sourcebook.* Chicago: Aldine, 1968.

Fuller, R. Buckminster. *Operating Manual for Spaceship Earth.* New York: Clarion, 1969.

Hall, A. D., & Fagen, R. E. Definition of a system. In Walter Buckley (ed.), *Modern Systems Research For the Behavioral Scientist: A Sourcebook.* Chicago: Aldine, 1968, pp. 81–92.

Litterer, Joseph (Ed.). *Organizations: Systems, Control and Adaptation: Vol. II, Second Edition.* New York: John Wiley, 1969.

Miller, James. Living systems: basic concepts. *Behavioral Science*, 1965, *10*, 93–237.

Miller, James. Living Systems, cross level hypotheses. *Behavioral Science*, 1965, *10*, 380–411.

Rapoport, Anatol. Foreword. In Walter Buckley (Ed.), *Modern Systems Research for the Behavioral Scientist: A Sourcebook.* Chicago: Aldine, 1968, pp. xiii–xxii.

Rogers, Martha. *An Introduction to the Theoretical Basis of Nursing.* Philadelphia: F. A. Davis, 1970.

Stern, Jess (Ed.). *The Random House Dictionary of the English Language:* The *Unabridged Edition.* New York: Random House, 1967.

Suttles, Gerald. *The Social Order of the Slum: Ethnicity and Territory in the Inner City.* Chicago: University of Chicago, 1970.

Warren, Roland. *The Community in America.* Chicago: Rand McNally, 1963.

Watts, Alan. *The Book: On the Taboo Against Knowing Who You Are.* New York: Vintage, 1966.

RESOURCES

Bates, Frederick, & Bacon, Lloyd. The community as a social system. *Mental Health Digest*, 1972, 4, 11–14.

Bertalanffy, Ludwig von. General system theory—A critical review. In Joseph Litterer (Ed.). *Organizations: Systems, Control and Adaptation.* (Second Edition.) Vol. II. New York: John Wiley, 1969, pp. 7–30.

Flagle, Charles. The role of simulation in the health services. *American Journal of Public Health.* 1970, *60*, 2386–2394.

Hearn, Gordon (Ed.). *The General Systems Approach: Contributions Toward an Holistic Conception of Social Work.* New York: Council on Social Work Education, 1969.

Hippocrates. Airs, waters, places. In John Chadwick and William Mann (Trans.). *The Medical Works of Hippocrates.* Oxford: Blackwell Scientific Publications, pp. 90–111. 1950.

Kandle, Roscoe. Report of the chairman of the technical development board to the governing council, 1959–1960. *American Journal of Public Health.* 1961, *51*, 287–294.

Laing, R. D. Intervention in social situations. In *The Politics of the Family and other Essays,* New York: Vintage, 1971.

McLuhan, Marshall, & Fiore, Quentin. *The Medium is the Massage.* New York: Bantam, 1967.

Wiener, Norbert. *The Human Use of Human Beings: Cybernetics and Society.* New York: Avon, 1954.

Wald, Lillian. *The House on Henry Street.* New York: Holt, Rinehart and Winston, 1915. (Reprinted, New York: Dover, 1971.)

2

PART TWO

Tools for Assessing Community Health

Concepts and principles related to health are presented for use in assessing the health of a community that you have identified as your system for study.

2

Chapter Two

Health, Community Health, and Community Health Assessment

Health—the sparkle, growth, and joy of living; *community*—people with a common bond; and *community health assessment*—the process of identifying both positive and negative forces in the health of a community: these are the basic notions in community health assessment.

Definitions

Health

Health is an elusive notion. Some definitions stress the lack of active disease processes. Others focus on degrees of independence in daily living (Burak, 1965). The most satisfactory ones emphasize self-actualization, the fulfilment of the individual, and the concept of high level wellness (Dunn, 1959, 1961; Maslow, 1971). Nancy Milio expressed her definition in poetry, "Health is wholeness, unfolding" (1970).

The basic components of any of the more satisfactory definitions of health are:

1. Energy—vitality, sparkle, *joie de vivre*
2. Individuality—uniqueness of the person that comes from the freedom to be and enjoy being oneself (Rogers, C., 1967)
3. Relationship—openness of the individual to himself and to others, relatedness, interaction (Rogers, C., 1967)
4. Development—the process of continuing growth (Milio, 1970)

The truly healthy person, alive and vital, seems to exude energy, to enjoy being himself. He enjoys relationships in which both he and others are free to be vital, sensitive to others, and uniquely themselves.

Community Health

Community health is a function of the energy, the individuality, and the relationships of the community as a whole, and of the individuals and groups within the community. The health of individuals is reflected in the health of the community, and the health of the community is reflected in the health of its people (Downs, 1974).

The sparkle, the life, the caring, the sense of direction and of enjoyment of life, the balance between growth and contentment within a community are some of the indicators of its overall wellness. Definitions of community health are few. There are many more measurable indicators of the ill health of a community than there are of its wellness. Flip your thinking around and, instead of looking at infant mortality, consider the percentage of children conceived who are born and who grow into productive maturity. This percentage is one indicator of a community's ability to function. Other indicators are the percentage of people who are employed (the community's ability to provide jobs to those who want them); the percentage of homes with heat and hot water (the community's ability to provide these basic necessities); the percentage of people who belong to some established primary group (belonging and loved); the percentage of people engaged in volunteer activities (altruism) (Maslow, 1962).

Any individual reflects a miniature picture of the forces which operate in his or her community. Successful resolution of developmental crises and commu-

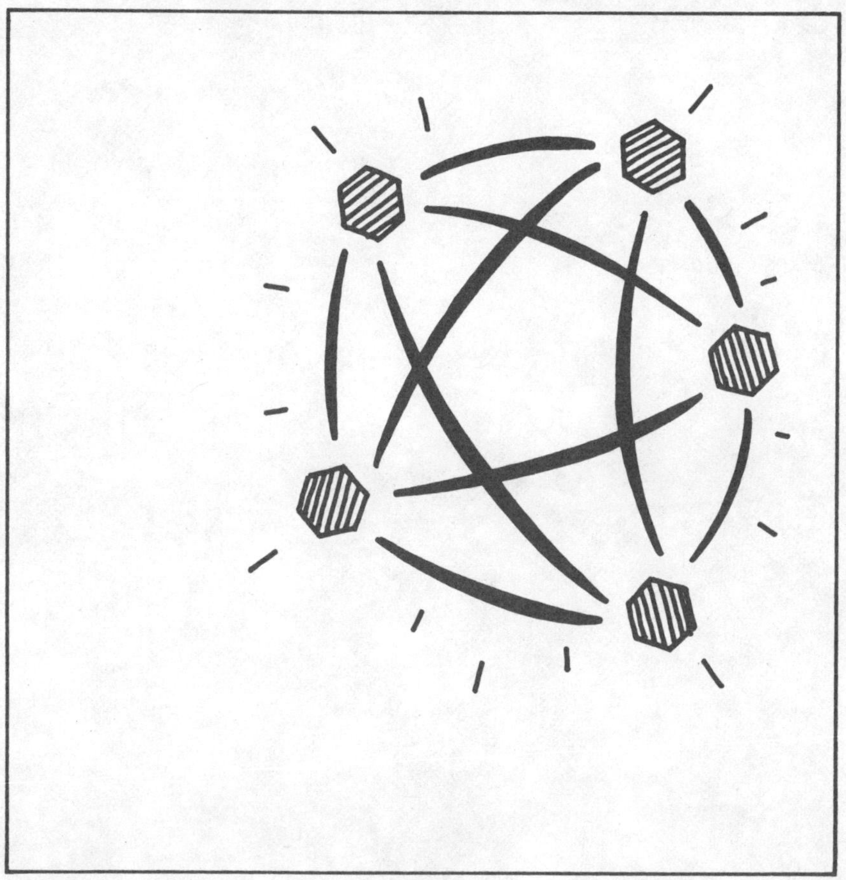

nity culture and resources for assisting individuals with each developmental phase are other indicators of the level of community health. The community's methods of dealing with its own developmental crises are a prime indicator of the wellness of the community as a whole.

Community Health Assessment

Community health assessment is the process of *defining* a community as a system, *identifying* the attributes of its components and describing the pattern and organization of the community in reference to its level of wellness.

How does the community deal with demands for its own growth? Coherently, logically, effectively or randomly, angrily, ineffectively? Watch the newspaper, for accounts of proposals for new roads, bridges, parks, or changes in the zoning laws to see how the community responds to growth.

References and Resources

REFERENCES

Burak, Bernard. Interdisciplinary classification for the aged. *Journal of Chronic Diseases,* 1965, *18,* 1059–1064.

Downs, Florence. Personal Communication. 1974.

Dunn, Halbert. *High Level Wellness.* Arlington, Va.: R. W. Beatty 1961.

Dunn, Halbert. High level wellness for man and society. *American Journal of Public Health,* 1959, 49, 786–792.

Maslow, Abraham. *The Farther Reaches of Human Nature.* New York: Viking, 1971.

Maslow, Abraham. *Toward a Psychology of Being.* Princeton: D. Van Nostrand, 1962.

Milio, Nancy. 9226 *Kercheval: The Storefront that Did Not Burn.* Ann Arbor: University of Michigan, 1970.

Rogers, Carl. Learning to be free. In Carl Rogers & Barry Stevens, *Person to Person: The Problem of Being Human: A New Trend in Psychology.* Lafayette, Calif.: Real People, 1967.

RESOURCES

Carlson, Gail & Irene Ruys-Nelson. *The Discovery of Human Potentials.* Madison Wisc.: Section of Child Behavior and Development, Bureau of Community Health Services, Division of Health, Department of Health & Social Services, 1971.

Goldsmith, Seth. The status of health status indicators. *Health Services Reports,* 1972, 87, 212–220.

Lynch, Kevin. *The Image of the City.* Cambridge, Mass.: MIT, 1960.

Northern Bolivar County Health & Civic Improvement Council, Inc. Good health is many things. Mound Bayou, Miss. (Printed flyer) n.d.

Rogers, Martha. *Introduction to a Theoretical Basis of Nursing.* Philadelphia: F. A. Davis, 1970.

Stern, Jess (Ed.) *The Random House Dictionary of the English Language: The Unabridged Edition.* New York: Random House, 1967.

Shuttles, Gerald. *The Social Order of the Slum: Ethnicity and Territory in the Inner City.* Chicago: University of Chicago, 1968.

U.S. Department of Health, Education, and Welfare; Public Health Service. *Conceptual Problems in Developing an Index of Health.* National Center for Health Statistics. Series 2, Number 17. (Public Health Service Publication No. 1000-Series 2-No. 17), May, 1966.

Warren, Roland. *The Community in America.* Chicago: Rand McNally, 1963.

Wooley, P. O., Hays, W. S., and Larson, D. L. *Syncrisis: The Dynamics of Health: An Analytic Series on the Interactions of Health and Socioeconomic Development. III. Perspectives and Methodology*, Washington, D.C.: U.S. Government Printing Office, June, 1972.

World Health Organization. *Measurement of Levels of Health: Report of a Study Group*, W.H.O. Technical Report Series #137. Geneva. W.H.O., 1957.

3

Chapter Three

Energy: Weighted and Unweighted Forces in Health

Energy, one of the components of our definition of health, is basic to community, to health, and to community health. There are many types of energy in the community and many attributes which can be used to describe these forms of energy. The distribution of energy is related both to its attributes and to the pattern and organization of the community. The attributes of energy which affect its distribution which will be considered in this chapter include: attractiveness, goal-directedness, amount, direction, distribution, and rhythms of energy flow.

Many of the concepts are presented as polarities (for example, open—closed; attractive—repulsive). This was done to provide a means of identifying specific attributes, which, in reality, are mixed in both type and degree. That is, the realities seen are the result of a variety of forces of differing degrees, all of which interact with the others in some way. Identifying the composition of each force provides a means of assessment that can serve as a basis for designing strategies for health.

Definitions

Health

Energy is power, the ability to do work (Stern, 1967). More accurately, the *flow* of energy is power (Logan, 1978). It can be actual, here-and-now energy or potential, yet-to-be-released energy (Miller, 1965, p. 193). Any living system requires energy to maintain its functions and to grow.

Community Health

The level of community health is dependent upon the adequacy of the many types of energies, both real and potential, within the community, and available to it in its environment, to perform those tasks which need to be accomplished.

The basic resource of a community, as of any living system, is energy, the capacity to do work.

People are the basic units of communities and are, in themselves, the basic energy of a community. Other energy sources and resources maintain, support, and provide the stimulus to growth of the people in the community. The energy level of the community as a whole is dependent upon the energy of its people. The energy of the people depends on the energy of the community. The community needs the energy of people to maintain its own functioning and to continue its development. The people need the community's functioning to maintain their own energy and to grow.

The functions of a community can be considered to be parallel to Maslow's (1955) hierarchy of need. A community provides for the following needs of its members:

1. Survival
2. Safety and security
3. Belonging, trust, and love
4. Altruism

Warren's (1963, pp. 9–10) description of the functions of community is very similar to this list. He considers the functions of a community to be:

1. Production-distribution-consumption
2. Socialization
3. Social control
4. Social participation
5. Mutual support

The energies of a community are required to maintain the functions of a community and to assist it in its own process of growth.

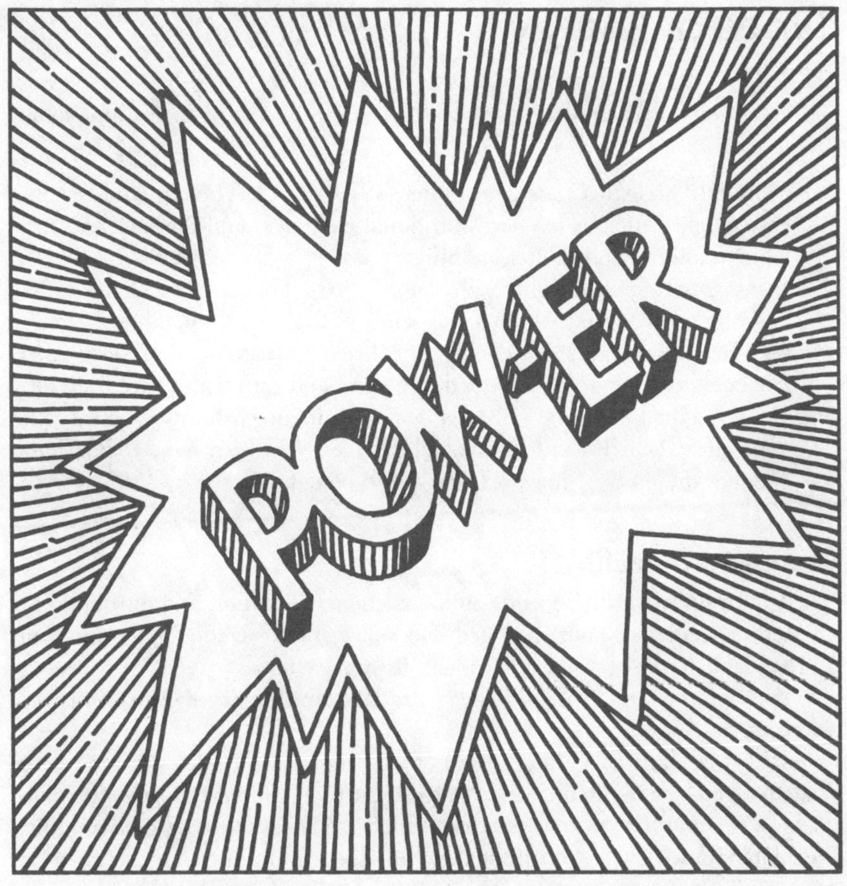

Community Health Assessment

What is the energy level of the community? Does it feel active or quiet? Do you feel energized by being there, relaxed, or drained of energy?

What tasks are being accomplished successfully? Are people clothed, sheltered, and fed adequately? Are they safe from accidents, fires, and violence? Do they (especially the older people) feel that they have an adequate vehicle for expression of their need to care for others?

Types of Energy

Health

The individual requires many types of energy to maintain his functioning and to grow.

1. *Material, "weighted" energies* (Fuller, 1970, p. 62). These include: chemical energies, such as oxygen, nutritional elements, and the materials from which clothing and shelter are built.
2. *Unweighted energies* (Fuller, 1970, pp. 61–62). These include: light, sound, and other wave forms which act as sensory stimuli. Information, awareness and the knowledge which enables effective action are another form. Affective energies such as love, hate, desire, fear, and caring provide a third form of unweighted energies. Other known and unknown forms of energy produce effects which can be described (Krieger, 1975; LeShan, 1974). These energies themselves, however, remain to be defined.

Community Health

Community health depends on the adequacy, amount, and distribution of all forms of energy—both weighted and unweighted—within the community and available to the community through its suprasystem.

Many forms and types of energy, are used and produced by and in communities.

Weighted energies (Fuller, 1970, p. 62) in communities are most often related to goods, and often closely related to survival and safety needs. Weighted energies include the natural resources which are accessible to the community, the materials which are distributed within the community and between the community and its suprasystem. Food, water, heating oil, and building materials are examples of "weighted" material energies.

Unweighted energies (Fuller, 1970, pp. 61–62) are more often related to services. The services provided by social agencies or by the people in the neighborhood who care (the "healers") are examples of unweighted energies. Information itself is unweighted, but it may or may not be bound to weighted carriers of that information, such as newspapers or posters. A television set (weighted) receives the unweighted signals which are sent by the transmitter (weighted). Word of mouth is unweighted.

Economic energies may be bound to material, weighted goods or to nonmaterial, unweighted services.

Physical, psychological, or psychic touch (Kreiger, 1975; Leshan, 1974; Rogers, C., 1967; Storm, 1972) carry unweighted healing energies which have yet to be fully defined.

The culture of a community is an unweighted energy, although it may be expressed in weighted forms—the relative size, number, and style of schools, churches, hospitals, theaters, playgrounds, and playground equipment (Stone & Rudolph, 1970).

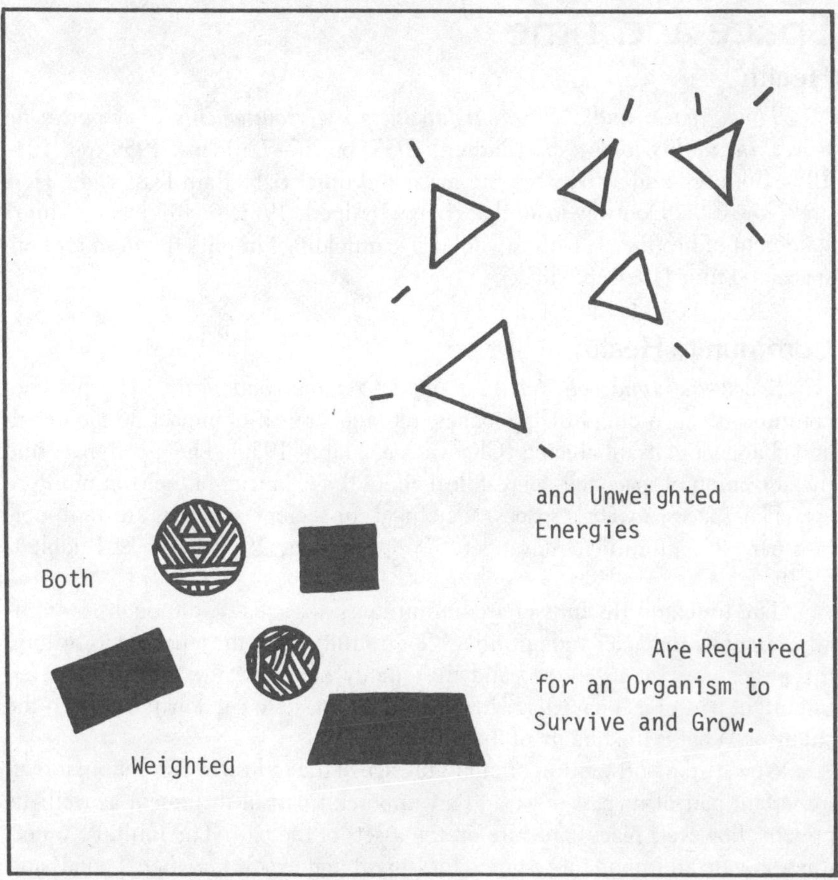
and Unweighted
Energies
Both
Are Required
for an Organism to
Survive and Grow.
Weighted

People are the basic units of communities. They are neither purely weighted nor unweighted as a form of energy, but something which results from the synergy of both material and nonmaterial energies. People provide the vitality (energy) of a community and, to a large degree, set the character of the community.

Community Health Assessment

What are the major energies in the community? What are the major resources for export? What are the major resources that have to be imported from the suprasystem? What is the apparent energy level of the people? Are most people young, vibrant, full of physical energy? Are older people with the fullness of knowledge and feeling that comes with experience? Is there a sense of caring and concern among the people? Are there many "healers," or few?

Space and Time

Health

Time, space, and their interrelatedness are requirements or resources for power, the ability to do work (Barnett, 1957, pp. 67–72; Joans, 1959, pp. 104–108). Both rest and activity require space and time. Baba Ram Dass said, "Here and Now is the Doorway to all that energy" (Alpert, 1971, p. 46). Nancy Milio's statement of health, "Health is wholeness, unfolding" implies the need for both space and time (1970, p. xiii).

Community Health

Space and time both have an impact on the community. The place of community, according to Hippocrates, has a great deal of impact on the health and character of its inhabitants (Chadwick & Mann, 1950). The use of space and the allocation of space tells a great deal about the character of the community.

Play spaces, meeting spaces, sociofugal, or sociopetal spaces are an important part of community (Alexander, 1968; Sommer, 1974; Stone & Rudolph, 1970).

The time and rhythms of a community speak equally, although less visually, about its character and priorities. Community time, the length of its history, the projections for its future, and the quality of each "now" are likewise an important part of its character. How long does it take to get downtown from the suburbs? What is the quality of that time?

New York's port was important in the age of the industrial revolution; it is an important part of its past now, and an important part of its present as well. Its present, however, places pressure on the assets of the past. The multiple waterways provide an important resource for import and export of material goods and of culture. But as technology advances, and more and more people depend on technology, technology depends upon more and more workers for survival and growth. New York's waterways—points of access during the industrial revolution—have become barriers to the entrance and exit of people who work, but do not live in the city.

The spaces and times of a community must be congruent with the needs of its people. Children require space to run, stretch their muscles and their voices. Young adults and middle-aged people require space for privacy, for exercise and recreation. Older people require all of the above and, in addition, quiet spaces to be with each other. All ages require space for privacy, exercise, meeting, and discussion (Chermayeff & Alexander, 1965).

Community time can facilitate access or establish barriers to resources. Evening store hours, blue laws, hours of darkness and of light, buildings which remain unused, HELP lines or HOT line hours can match or mismatch the hours in which the relevant services are required. Bus lines that do not carry people to the emergency room on Sundays or during late night hours may mismatch the need.

The pace of community—the speed with which people move through its

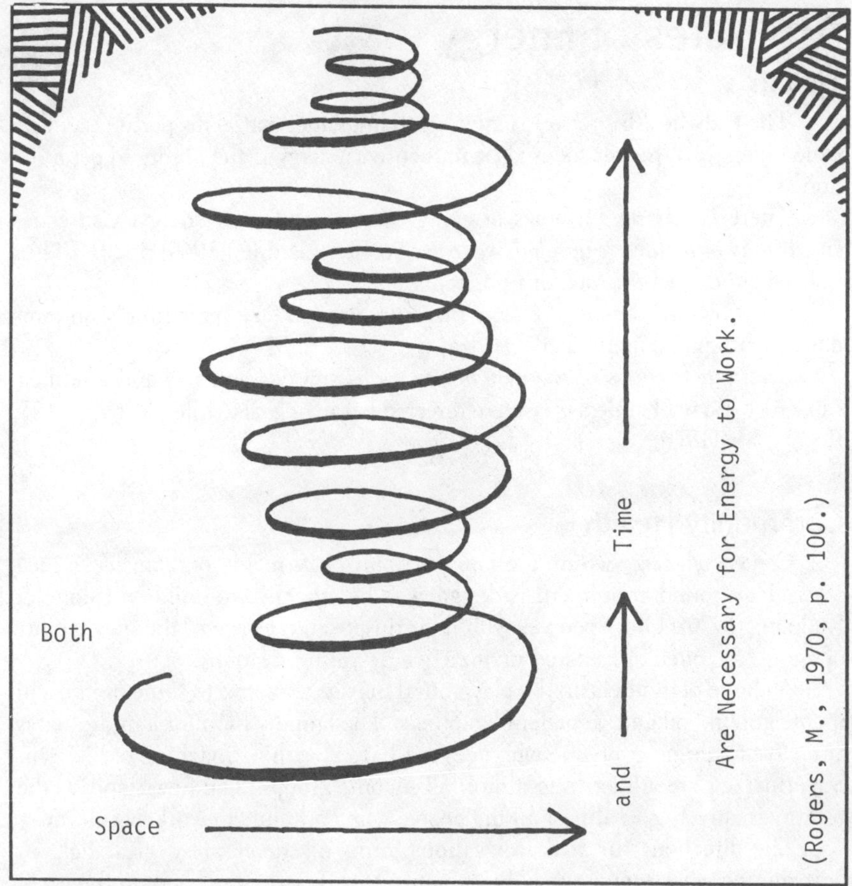
Both
Space
and
Time
Are Necessary for Energy to Work.
(Rogers, M., 1970, p. 100.)

spaces—adds another dimension to the understanding of a community's unique character.

The sense of space and the use of space in community varies greatly. The constricted spaces of Manhattan are in great contrast to the expansive spaces of the Midwest. A community hemmed in by mountains provides a different environment than one set in the middle of a plain. A community with easy access to the outdoors and dramatic seasonal changes provides a very different environment than one where seasons come and go with little more impact on the senses than a change in temperature.

Community Health Assessment

What is the sense of place—expansive, open, contracted, or closed? What is the sense of time—hurried or slow? What are the high points of the community's history? What are the spatial barriers between segments of the community—the proverbial tracks which divide? What does the community's history provide to its sense of identity? To what degree is the community in synchronization with its time and place? To what degree does it deny these, and in what ways?

Attributes of Energy

Health

The truly healthy person is alive, sparkling, and vital. This person seems to exude energy. Whether focused or unfocused, energy is the ability to get a job done.

There are many attributes of energy and of centers of energy. *Centers of energy may be attractive or repulsive to each other.* (Gardner, 1969, p. 201). They may be either goal-directed or undirected.

Goal-directed centers of energy (negentropic) produce increasingly nonrandom, or unique, patterned effects.

Undirected centers of energy (entropic) tend toward sameness and lose their capacity to do work unless they are redirected toward a goal (Miller, 1965, p. 195; Rogers, M., 1970).

Community Health

Centers of energy within a community may be attractive or repulsive to each other. Playground equipment is designed to be attractive to children (Stone & Rudolph, 1970). Older people, with their unspoken message of the inevitability of aging, are often considered unattractive by younger groups.

A clique of mothers on the playground may be attractive to some mothers in the neighborhood and "repellent" to others. The laundry room or laundromat is attractive to almost everyone who does not have a washing machine of his own. Supermarkets are attractive to almost all income groups. The newsstand by the subway is attractive to almost all the people who commute to work by subway.

The directions, or goals, of various forms of energy are a great help in determining what energies may be attractive to different groups within the community (Alinsky, 1969). The people who are interested in maintaining the playground are almost inevitably attracted to those who want to save their apartment building, when both are facing the task of stopping the construction of a highway which is planned to pass through both areas.

The health of communities depends upon the ability of individuals and groups within the community to work toward common goals. It does not require that all hold the same goals, nor that all groups work toward the same goals at all times. It does require, however, that all groups do work together toward the same goal at the same time when they are faced with a real survival threat to the community (such as occurs in the face of a natural disaster, or a technological disaster like the East Coast blackout of 1965). It does require that all interested subsystems of the community can work toward the same goal when it is relevant to their needs. The department of parks should be able to work with the board of education if both are interested in setting up an evening and weekend recreation program on the school playground. It would be even better if the P.T.A., the mothers of preschool children, and the older people who live in the neighborhood could also be sufficiently attracted to a meeting to plan the program. One

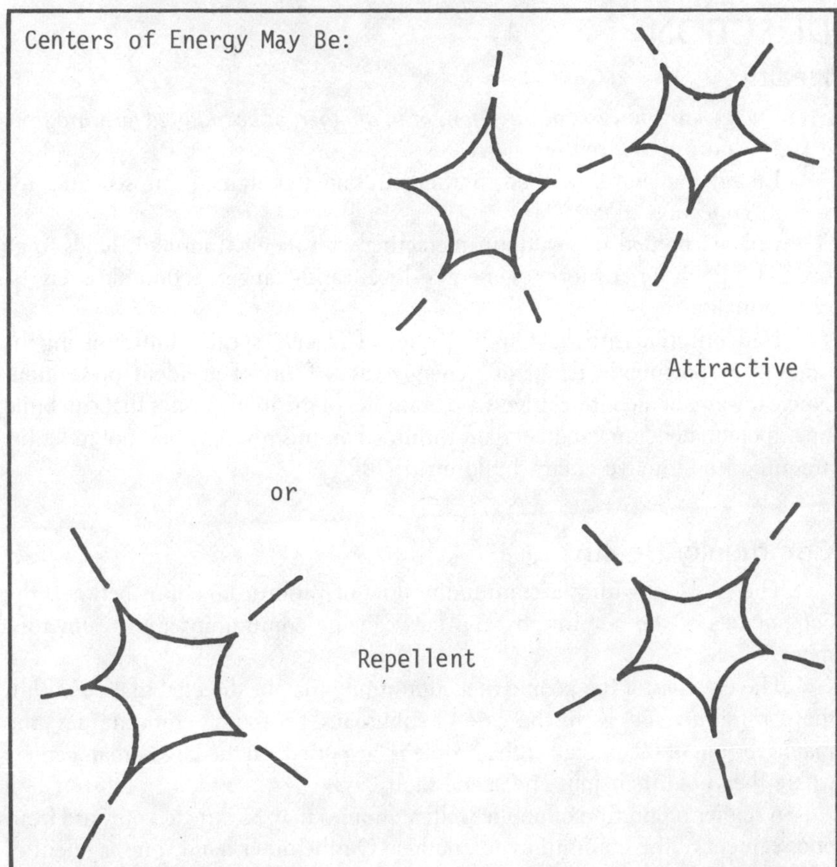
Centers of Energy May Be:
Attractive
or
Repellent

would have to locate the energy sources which were attractive to each of these groups in order to provide the information about the meeting and its goals.

Community Health Assessment

What groups in the community hold common or near-common goals? Are they in fact attracted by each other? What groups hold similar goals? Do they appear to be attracted by each other? If not, what are the "repelling" factors? Are there conflicting needs for the same limited resources? Are there different beliefs about methods of achieving goals? What groups in the community are "repelled" by each other? Are there any common areas of attraction?

What energy centers in the community are attractive to what groups of people?

Is there sense or evidence that a preponderance of attractive or repellent energy centers exist within the community?

DIRECTION

Health

Energy may flow in one direction, or in another, or be radiated outward from or drawn inward to a central source.

Energy may not flow at all, but remain static, contained, unused, in some sort of "collection center."

Energy, bottled up, without interacting with its environment, tends to go bad. This holds for any form of energy—love, caring, anger, economic energies, or information.

Haddon, in his article "On the Escape of Tigers," speaks of minimizing the buildup of potentially dangerous energies as a form of accident prevention. Nuclear waste or alcoholic drivers are examples of the many things that can build up as potentially damaging energies within a community. It is best not to let the amount of destructive energy build up (1970).

Community Health

The energies within a community flow in various directions between the components of the community and between the community and its environment.

The energies of the people in a community may be directed to tasks within the community, or, as in the case of suburban "bedroom" communities, the major portion of the energy of the people is "exported" to the large urban centers where they hold their jobs and spend their days.

A higher proportion of public welfare monies may be directed outward from one segment of the community to another. On the other hand, one segment of the community may import (draw in) human energies in the form of skills or service jobs. If these are paid for, a certain amount of economic energy flows out from the employer. It may or may not be proportionate to the imported energies.

The pulse of energy inflow and outflow can be seen in the media, where information is gathered (imported) by the news media for the purpose of dissemination (export) in order to make money (import).

A *balance of energy flow is required for community health.* Communities that depend heavily on imported energies, from few sources, are vulnerable to these sources. Communities that export more resources than they import are a high risk for decay. Most of the cooperative movement and the struggle of the 1960's was based on the awareness that no community could afford to export more economic resources than it took in itself (Comprehensive Manpower, 1973). Food cooperatives provide a way to minimize the export of economic energies to corporations outside of the community. Credit unions operate on the same principle, favoring people who belong to the credit union in the local area.

The public health nurse making home visits is carrying resources (energies) of information and caring outward from her agency to the homes of her clients. The clinic brings the energies (positive and negative) of people and their health problems inward to its center.

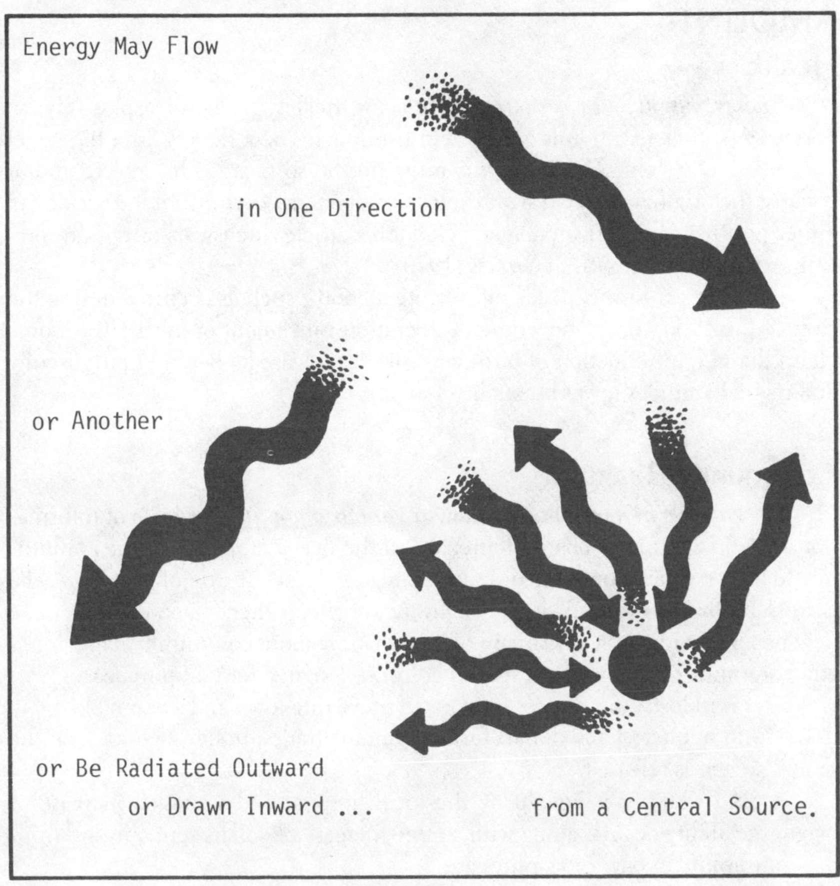
Energy May Flow
in One Direction
or Another
or Be Radiated Outward
or Drawn Inward ...
from a Central Source.

Community participation in health care planning was established in order to get information regarding health needs from the consumers to the providers of care. This has not always worked. The focus has often been on informing consumers about the constraints on the providers of medical care services.

Community Health Assessment

What energies does the community depend upon most heavily for import? What is the cost in terms of energies that must be exported to obtain them?

How many stores are locally owned? Where do the bulk of taxes come from? (Sales taxes? If so, what items are included—soaps, clothing, paper products?) Real estate taxes? Where are these taxes paid to? In what directions do these dollars flow? Do they go upward to still higher levels of government, or back to the community (See Warren, 1963, on horizontal and vertical relationships, pp. 237–302). For what purposes are they used? In which directions do what energies flow within the community?

AMOUNT

Health

Energy may flow in various amounts, in trickles, rivers, or explosively, in booms. A sufficient amount of energy must flow to meet the needs of the target system or subsystem. However, this must not be so great as to deplete and/or exhaust the original source. Great explosions of energy occur from the backlog of either positive or negative energies. Haddon's article discusses strategies to prevent explosions of negative energies (1970).

A backlog of unmet needs may create a boom, such as occurred during the riots of the 1960's or in the women's liberation movement of the 1970's. Some claim that the introduction of birth control pills released a boom of promiscuity and revised attitudes toward sexuality.

Community Health

The energies in a community flow in various amounts. A trickle of information may flow from the board of directors of the major employer in the community to the newspaper or to the union members. A steady stream of people may be carried by the bus system or the highway system to their place of work. The newspaper provides a steady stream of information about community happenings and community meetings in a special column designed for that purpose.

A new industry announces its plans to move into town and a boom of energy in the form of interest and dollars for the building trades, or new demands on the school system is released.

A CAT scanner is bought by the local hospital and a sudden increase of diagnostic ability occurs, along with a large increase of dollars sent outward from the community to pay for its purchase.

The chemical energies required for nutrition flow in trickles in economically depressed areas. The farmer who has one chicken, gets only one egg a day for protein. Large rivers of protein flow from the supermarket to the "average American family" in the "average American city."

Programs such as Meals on Wheels and nutritional programs for women, infants, and children are planned to enlarge the flow of nutritional energies to members of the community.

Community health depends upon an adequate distribution of energies to all members (individuals or groups) within the community, and between the community and its suprasystem.

The amount of any form of energy which flows within a community must be balanced between the resources of the originating source and the need of its target. Adequacy and appropriateness of amounts of energy become increasingly relevant in an era of scarcity such as the present one. The oil embargo provides a classic example of a form of energy decreasing to a trickle, and thereby hampering the community in its distribution of other forms of energy. People had great difficulty getting to work. Much time was spent waiting in line for gas. The

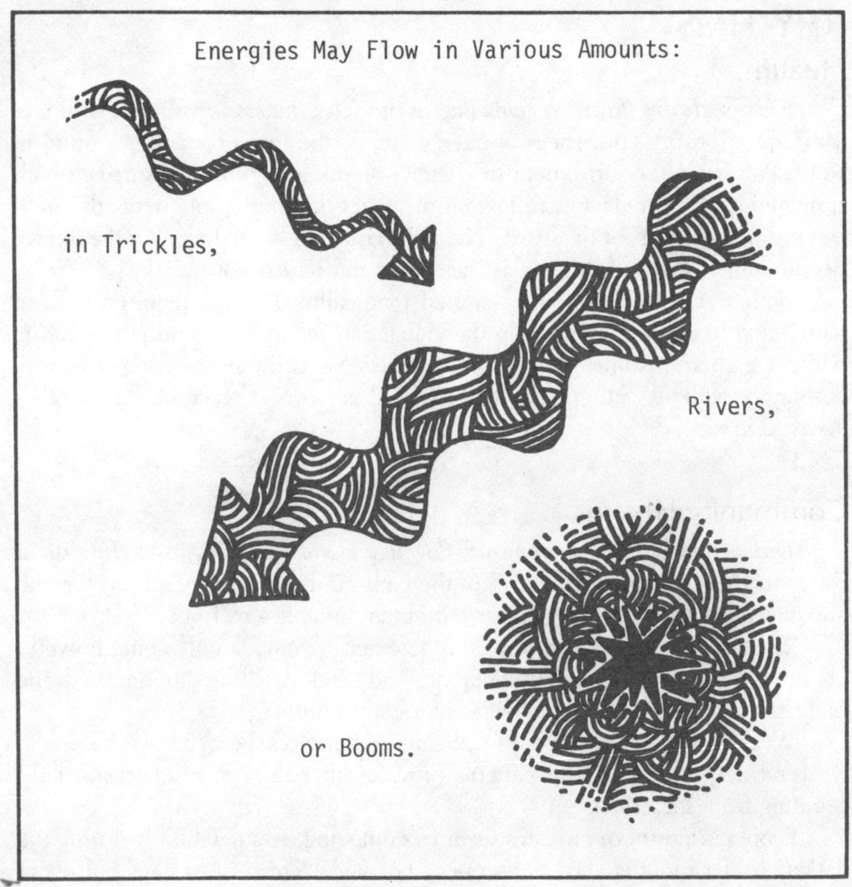
Energies May Flow in Various Amounts:
in Trickles,
Rivers,
or Booms.

energies syphoned off to solve the problem of getting gas depleted the amount of human energy available to the community for other purposes.

Bits of information about legislation for national health insurance in the United States are provided by the media. Those interested and involved in health care legislation must maintain contact with their legislators to give them the information necessary to legislate for their needs.

Community Health Assessment

Where would a health worker find access to a steady stream of information about the health needs of a community? Where are the areas of imbalance between the energy source, the needs of its targets, and the amount of energy that flows between them? What is your best guess for the next cultural, attitudinal, or value explosion in your community? Try looking for the greatest backlog of unexpressed feeling or need as your first clue.

RHYTHMS

Health

Energy always flows, to some degree in cycles, pulses, or waves (Murchie, 1967, pp. 366 ff.) The spaces of energy are, as the space of matter, bound in time. Pulses are the movement of energies across space and measured in both time and space. An electrocardiogram measures the motion of energy throughout the areas (spaces) of the heart. The most visible pulse of the city is the flow of people into and out of the city as they go to and return from work.

Both rest and activity are required for health. Time is required both to gather and to expend energy. No individual can maintain the output of caring without gathering some rewards for himself. No community group can give constantly without gathering either material resources, recognition, or other assets to itself.

Community Health

The energies within a community flow in a cyclical fashion, just as they do in the individual. Circadian rhythms of the community can be seen from the ebb and flow of people on a street corner at different times of day (Luce, 1971, p. 40).

The hustle and bustle of the commerce of the day, people going to work, children to school, housewives shopping, and vendors selling, contrast with the night people and nighttime activities in a community.

Weekly patterns include the obvious differences between weekday and weekend activities. Seasonal patterns provide differences in climate and tasks resulting from the climate.

People in northern climates seem less outgoing, less neighborly during the darker, colder months and, as one neighbor said, "creep from their burrow at work and back to their burrow at home without looking in either direction." Alcoholism and suicide rates in dark northern climates are higher than those in warm, sunny southern climates. Children play less on playgrounds, mothers meet less while watching them and neighbors are not inclined to stop and talk on the sidewalk when it is 20 degrees below zero. The flow of caring energies seems drawn in by the energy demands for warmth and security.

Some activity is required at all times to maintain the life of the community. The night workers who monitor and maintain necessary community functions may need to adapt their individual day and night cycles to the needs of the community as a whole. Night workers in the hospital, in the police and fire departments, bus or cab drivers, clerks in the all-night delicatessen, workers at the radio or TV station that reaches those who cannot or will not sleep, all support a minimal level of function for the needs of the community.

The need for a balance of energy flow across the seasons exists as well. Higher demands for health services may be present in the winter months. Seasonal industries draw into town migrant workers, be they affluent ski instructors

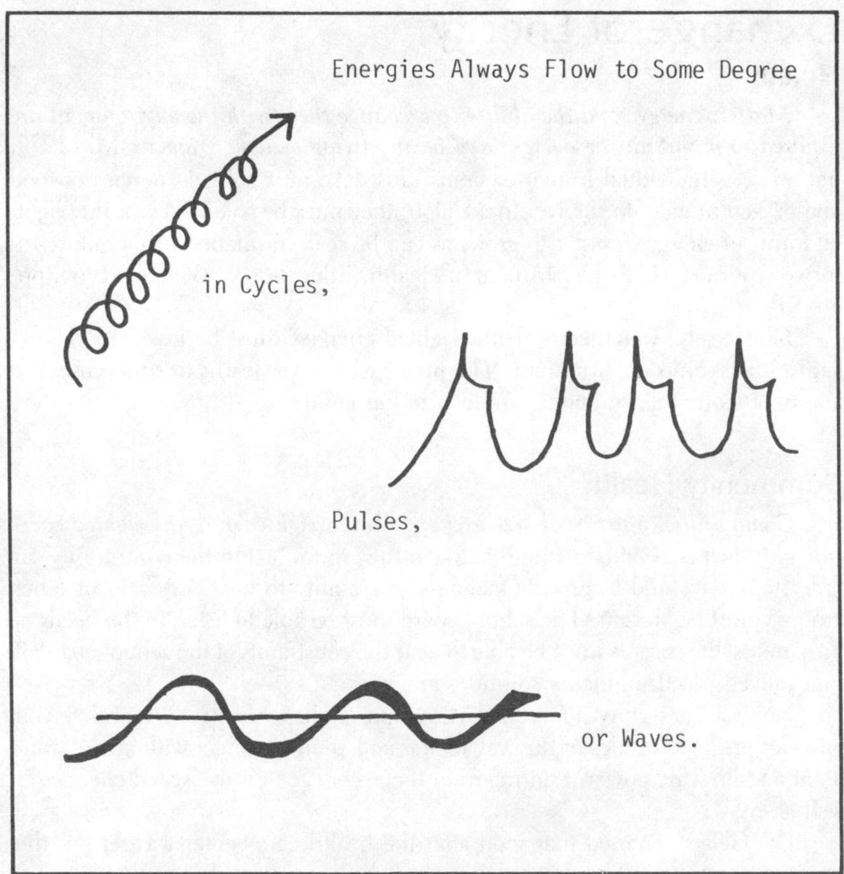
Energies Always Flow to Some Degree
in Cycles,
Pulses,
or Waves.

or impoverished fruit pickers. Many demands are placed on the community by seasonal industries such as education, skiing or sunning, and agriculture. The uneven ebb and flow of people places high demands on community resources such as schools, housing, restaurants, and health services.

Community Health Assessment

Stand on a corner for fifteen minutes and take its "vital signs" at four different times of day. How many people go by? Who are they? Are they old people, young people, or a mixture of both? Where are the children? Where are the older people? If you don't see them, why don't you? Does night belong to the deviants? (What does this tell you about the tolerance of the day people for deviance in themselves as well as in others?) What are the seasonal rhythms in your community?

Exchange of Energy

Health

Matter, energy, and the ability to exchange them with the environment are required to maintain the energy level of any living system. (Rogers, M., 1970, pp. 49–54). Individual human systems must take in weighted energies of food and oxygen in order to survive. In addition, they must be able to accept unweighted forms of energy in order to grow, as can be seen in infants with a failure-to-thrive syndrome (U.S. Department of Health, Education & Welfare, 1968, pp. 56–59).

Conversely, weighted and unweighted energies must be given by the organism back to its environment. The infant who never learns to smile loses the ability of its mother to cuddle and coo to her child.

Community Health

Communities must be able to exchange both weighted and unweighted energies with their environments, and between the groups within the community, in order to survive and to grow. Openness, the ability to hear messages of other groups, must be present. The school board must be able to listen to the needs of the parents; the parents must be able to hear the constraints of the school board; if innovative, growth-inducing solutions are to occur.

Jack Geiger's story about the Mississippi Delta project at Mound Bayou provides prime examples of the way matter and energy interact with an environment and how the power resulting from the exchange of unweighted energies as well (1969).

Dr. Geiger reported that soon after the health care center was set up, the people came to say "Thank you—It really is a fine center—but we are hungry, could you share some food with us?" With this exchange of information, rooted in a previous exchange of caring and sensitivity, the center began to stock food in its pharmacy as a specific treatment for malnutrition. Sometime later, the suggestion was made, "Why not start a garden club for those people who like to grow things." (Now we will jump ahead of ourselves to individuality, which is its own kind of energy.) So they put up a sign, asking people to come to a meeting about starting a garden club. "Well," says Dr. Geiger, "just about the whole community showed up." It seemed that all the people really liked to grow things. There was land nearby which was under government subsidy not to be used. Some exchanges with the suprasystem occurred, and the land was freed to be used by the people to grow crops. Soon they were growing more than they needed to feed themselves. The "Geiger formula" of putting things together that belong together—the energies of people who are hungry and who like to grow things; the rich Delta soil available to be cultivated; an atmosphere of listening and hearing, sensitivity, and sufficient concern—incorporates all the elements of human energies (weighted and unweighted) in interchange with each other toward the increased health of one community.

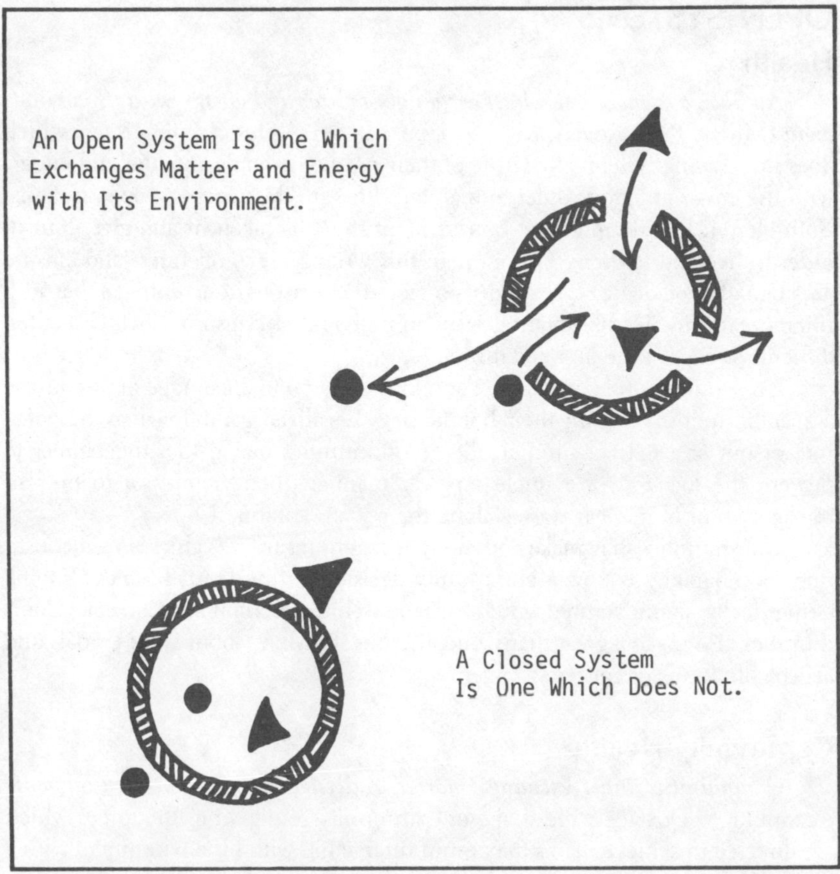
An Open System Is One Which
Exchanges Matter and Energy
with Its Environment.
A Closed System
Is One Which Does Not.

Community Health Assessment

What are the areas of greatest energy exchange between groups within the community? What are the areas of greatest energy exchange between the community and its suprasystem?

Is there freedom to express openness and caring between community groups? What groups in the community are the most open to listen to the needs of individual community members or of groups within the community? What groups within the community are most open to hear the health needs of all groups within the community? Which are most open to hear the needs of the groups within the community that most closely represent your area of interest?

OPEN SYSTEMS

Health

An open system is one which exchanges matter and energy with its environment (Miller, 1965; Rogers, M., 1970, pp. 49–54). A closed system is one which does not. Living systems, by virtue of their need to exchange matter and energy with the environment in order to maintain life, are, by necessity, open systems. Both chemical and emotional nourishment must be taken in and given out in order to live and to grow. However, in this writer's view, openness and closure are a matter of degree. The skin protects the person from entry of harmful microorganisms. Denial might protect an individual from stimuli which are too difficult to experience at a certain moment.

Communities may make the conscious decision to encourage or discourage a specific industry within their boundaries. Legalized gambling may be voted into or out of a state or municipality. Communities may gather their forces to prevent the location of a nuclear power plant in their vicinity or to prevent transportation of nuclear wastes along their roads (Braun, 1977).

Communities may make conscious decisions regarding values. What constitutes pornography is now a community decision in the United States. Buying domestically manufactured goods is a conscious decision in Canada. Communities also make a great many unconscious decisions about values, goals and acceptable forms of caring or anger.

Community Health

Communities must exchange matter and energy with their environment. According to Doxiades, the shape of community results from the forces which are directed to achieve man's maximum interaction with his environment with a minimum of expenditure of effort (1970).

Community, by its very essence, requires the ability of individuals and groups to give and take goods, services, goals, values, and ideals. In addition, the community must be in contact with material and nonmaterial goods from sources outside itself. Some communities attempt, or have attempted, to achieve near closure to outside influences, but absolute closure is impossible. Some import or export is required, and with that comes contact and consequent exchange of values and ideas.

Some political systems attempt closure by censoring the content of written or verbal communication and travel of the members of their community. Human tendencies for growth, new ideas, increased freedom, create an underground, striving for greater openness of information.

The concept of opening up health care planning to information from community members was pushed forward in the 1960's with the local community control of health care centers and requirements for community members on boards of local hospital and health care centers. The original intent was to obtain information from the members of the community regarding their needs for service. The emphasis soon changed to that of the need to educate consumers to

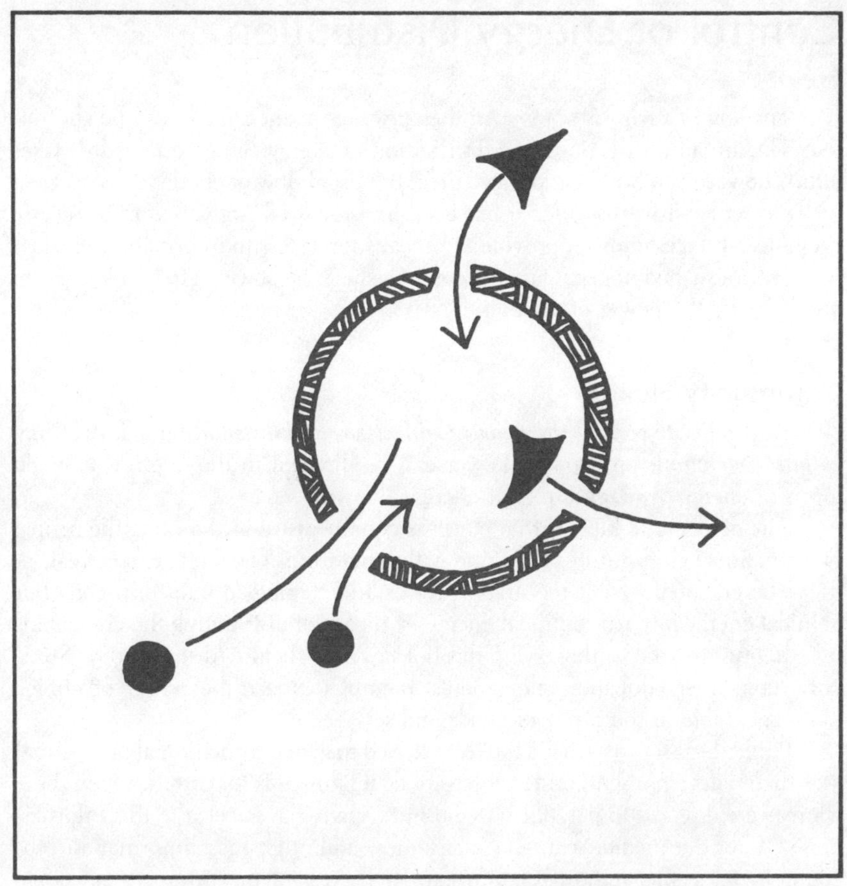

the jargon, values, and style of the planners. The community members' style, stronger in communication of feelings and values, seemed often to be the major bone of contention. Many of the works cited in support of inclusion of community members in planning were related to just this, the need for sensitivity in planning care (Humphries, 1971). Anger, however, was not bargained for, and certainly was not included in the traditional consumer role. The consumers of health care were still expected to express their gratitude. The only space left for their expression of anger was through the courts, and the denial of the opportunity to express this valid form of energy while in the patient role created a backlog of negative energy which could only be aired through the courts.

Community Health Assessment

What feelings can be expressed most openly in the community? Which ones are controlled, and which are suppressed? How are those which are suppressed vented? What are the community's labelled deviants saying about feelings and other energies which are not equally distributed within the community?

Control of Energy Distribution

Health

The flow of energy is power. All the attributes of energy flow can be controlled. The amount, direction, and distribution of energy can be directed. It takes effort, however, to build, stop, or redirect the usual flow of energy. It takes great effort to reestablish trust once it has been broken. It takes great effort to reverse prejudice. It takes effort to provide the means for access to information to those who previously had none. It takes energy to reduce the power vested in one group and increase the power of another.

Community Health

The ability to control the amount, direction, and distribution of any energy within a community is power. Power can be directed to the control of single forms of energy or many forms of energy.

The democratic ideal is that power is equally distributed among the people of the national community. Power, as with other forms of energy, can be real, or it can be potential. Voter registration drives are attempts to transform *potential* political energy into *real* political energy by means of distributing the credentials (registration) to vote to those who did not have this before (distribution). Similarly, consumer education movements attempt to make the power of choice more accessible to the buyer of goods and services.

Public health nurses have for years strived to give information about normal growth and development, and methods of facilitating this to parents. Often these efforts were directed to parents who did not usually have access to this information. Use of the media, women's magazines, and other mass information programs increase the amount of information flow, and the numbers of people reached. These people can then make informed choices about the behaviors and approaches they wish to pursue.

The direction of health dollars (economic energies) to "health purposes" may be controlled by health care planners rather than by consumers. A swimming pool may be considered as a health resource in a community. It provides recreation, socializing, and physical exercise, which result in increased sophistication of body concept and improved self image (Fisher & Cleveland, 1968). Health care planners might well exclude the pool from the definition of "health" on the basis that it provides no jobs for health workers or dollars for "health" facilities. The ability to control that decision is power.

Distribution of medical care resources, higher in the higher economic areas, lower in poor urban and rural areas, is considered a problem of national priority at this time. The trickle of medical care resources to rural areas and the lack of a physician in other areas constitute a problem in many countries. Senator Leahy (D., Vermont) in setting up hearings on rural health care, encouraged the distribution of information by holding hearings in Vermont as well

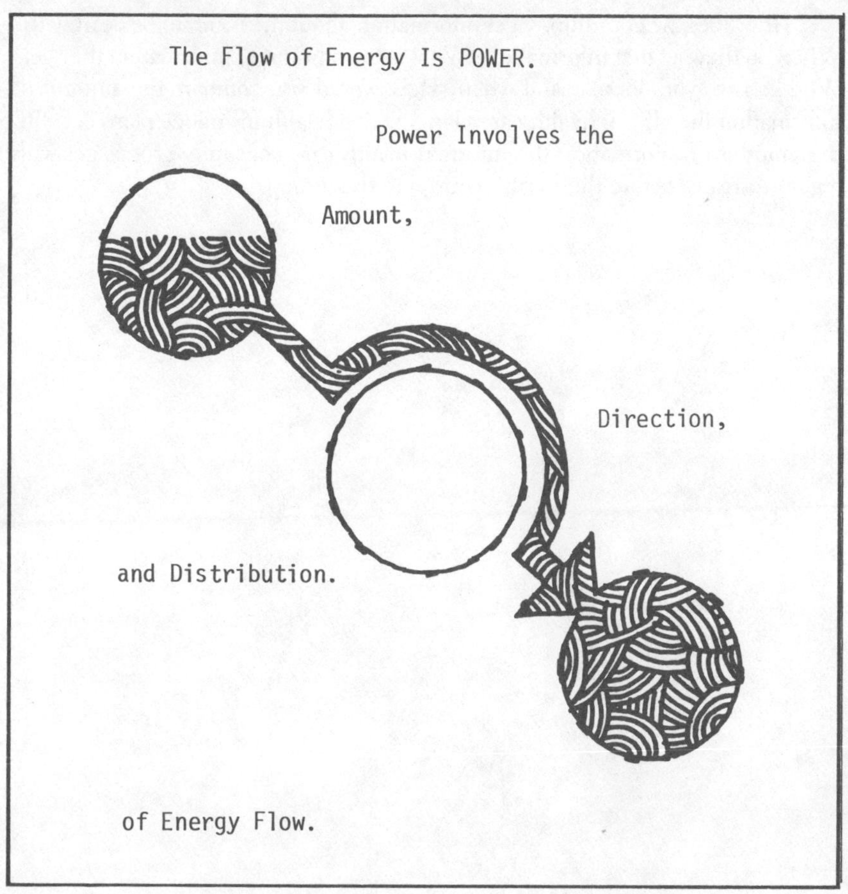
The Flow of Energy Is POWER.
Power Involves the
Amount,
Direction,
and Distribution.
of Energy Flow.

as in Washington (Senate Committee on Agriculture and Forestry, 1976). As a result, many more people were able to testify and to hear the testimony given than would have been possible if the hearings had been held only in Washington, D.C.

Community Health Assessment

Who participates in important decision-making in the community? Is it always the same few people? How are they accountable to others, and to the community at large? What is the proportion of people registered to vote? What are the relative proportions of people registered to vote in different sections of the community?

How are decisions about health care planning made? Who are the community representatives? How accessible and how accountable are they to the community? Are their positions on the issues accessible to the community?

How does the community get information about the issues to be dealt with? When do they get that information? What is the amount of information they get? Who gets it, who doesn't, and when? How would you compare the amount of information the official health care planners and health insurance plans get with the amount of information the informal health care consumer groups get with regard to issues before the local health planning group?

References and Resources

REFERENCES

Alexander, Christopher, Ishikawa, Sara, & Silverstein, Murray. *A Pattern Language Which Generates Multi-Service Centers.* Berkeley, Calif.: Center for Environmental Structure, 1968.

Alinsky, Saul. *Reveille for Radicals.* New York: Vintage, 1969.

Alpert, Richard (Baba Ram Dass). *Remember Be Here Now.* New York: Crown, 1971.

Barnett, Lincoln. *The Universe and Dr. Einstein.* New York: Bantam, 1957.

Braun, Bill. Vermonters resist nuclear power. *The Burlington Free Press,* March 2, 1977, p. 1.

Chermayeff, Serge & Alexander, Christopher. *Community and Privacy.* Garden City: Anchor, 1965.

Comprehensive manpower. *Restoration,* 3, July 1973. (Published by Bedford-Stuyvesant Restoration Corporation, New York).

Doxiades, Constantinos. Ekistics, the science of human settlements. *Science,* 1970, *170,* 394–404.

Fisher, Seymour & Cleveland, S. E. *Body Image and Personality.* (Revised Edition.) New York: Dover, 1968.

Fuller, R. Buckminster. *Operating Manual for Spaceship Earth.* New York: Clarion, 1969.

Gardner, Martin. *The Ambidextrous Universe: Left, Right, and the Fall of Parity.* New York: Mentor, 1969.

Geiger, H. Jack. The endlessly revolving door. *American Journal of Nursing,* 1969, *69,* 2436–2445.

Haddon, William. On the escape of tigers: an ecologic note. *American Journal of Public Health,* 1970, *60,* 2229–2234.

Hippocrates. Airs, Waters and Places. In John Chadwick and William Mann (Trans.), The Medical Works of Hippocrates. Oxford: Blackwell Scientific Publications, 1950, pp. 90–111.

Humphries, Mattie. Planning to heal the nation. *Public Administration Review,* 1971, *31,* 374–382.

Jeans, Sir James. *The New Background of Science.* Ann Arbor: University of Michigan, 1959.

Krieger, Dolores. Therapeutic touch: the imprimatur of nursing. *American Journal of Nursing,* 1975, *75,* 784–787.

LeShan, Lawrence. *The Medium, the Mystic and the Physicist: Toward a General Theory of the Paranormal.* New York: Viking, 1974.

Logan, Robert. Personal Communication. January 25, 1978.

Luce, Gay. Understanding body time in the 24-hour city. *New York*, November 15, 1971, pp. 38–43.

Maslow, Abraham. Deficiency motivation and growth motivation. In Marshall Jones (Ed.), *Nebraska Symposium on Motivation*, 3, 1–30. Lincoln: University of Nebraska, 1955.

Milio, Nancy. *9226 Kercheval: The Storefront that Did Not Burn*. Ann Arbor: University of Michigan, 1970.

Miller, James. Living Systems: Basic Concepts. *Behavioral Science*, 1965, *10*, 193–237.

Murchie, Guy. *Music of the Spheres: The Material Universe—From Atom to Quasar, Simply Explained. Vol. II. The Microcosm: Matter, Atoms, Waves, Radiation, Relativity*. New York: Dover, 1967.

Rogers, Carl. Learning to be free. In Carl Rogers & Barry Stevens, *Person to Person: The Problem of Being Human: A New Trend in Psychology*. Lafayette, Calif.: Real People Press, 1967, pp. 47–66.

Rogers, Martha. *An Introduction to the Theoretical Basis of Nursing*. Philadelphia: F. A. Davis, 1970.

Senate Committee on Agriculture and Forestry. *Success Stories in Rural Health Care delivery: Hearing Before the Subcommittee on Rural Development of the Committee on Agriculture and Forestry, United States Senate, Ninety-fourth Congress, Second Session*. Washington, D.C.: U.S. Government Printing Office, 1976.

Sommer, Robert. Our Airports are sociofugal, not sociopetal, and it's an outrage. *New York Times*, March 3, 1974, Section 10, pp. 1, 14, 15.

Stern, Jess (Ed.). *The Random House Dictionary of the English Language: The Unabridged Edition*. New York: Random House, 1967.

Stone, Jeanette & Rudolph, Nancy. *Play and Playgrounds*. Washington, D.C.: National Association for the Education of Young Children, 1970.

Storm, Hyemeyohsts. *Seven Arrows*. New York: Harper & Row, 1972.

U.S. Department of Health, Education and Welfare; Public Health Service; National Institutes of Health; The National Institute of Child Health and Human Development. *Perspectives on Human Deprivation: Biological, Psychological and Sociological*. Washington, D.C.: U.S. Government Printing Office, 1968.

Warren, Roland. *The Community in America*. Chicago: Rand McNally, 1963.

RESOURCES

Arnstein, Sherry. A ladder of citizen participation. *Journal of the American Institute of Planners*, 1969, 35, 216–224.

Bennis, Warren, Benne, Kenneth, & Chin, Robert (Eds.). *The Planning of Change*. New York: Holt, Rinehart & Winston, 1969.

Capra, Fritjof. *The Tau of Physics: An Exploration of the Parallels Between Modern Physics and Eastern Mysticism*. Berkeley, Calif.: Shambala, 1975.

Chermayeff, Serge & Tzionis, Alexander. *Shape of Community: Realization of Human Potential*. Baltimore: Penguin, 1971.

Christakis, George (Ed.). Nutritional assessment in health programs. *American Journal of Public Health*, 1973, *63*. (Supplement to November, 1973 issue.)

Dalton, Melville. Formal and informal organization. In Amatai Etzioni (Ed.), *Readings on Modern Organizations*. Englewood Cliffs, N.J.: Prentice-Hall, 1969, pp. 114–121.

Green, Elmer, Green, Alyce, & Walters, E. Dale. Biofeedback for mind-body self-regulation: Healing and Creativity. *Fields within Fields . . . Within Fields: The Methodology of Pattern*, 6, 131–144. New York: The World Institute Council, 1972.

Hall, Edward. *Beyond Culture*. Garden City: Anchor, 1977.

Halprin, Lawrence. *The RSVP Cycles: Creative Processes in the Human Environment*. New York: George Braziller, 1969.

Kuper, Hilda. The Language of sites in the politics of space. *American Anthropologist*. 1972, *74*, 411–425.

Laing, R. D. *The Politics of the Family and Other Essays*. New York: Vintage, 1972.

Lalonde, Marc. *A New Perspective on the Health of Canadians: A Working Document*. Ottawa: Government of Canada, April, 1974.

Latham, Michael & Cobos, Francisco. The effects of malnutrition on intellectual development and learning. *American Journal of Public Health*, 1971, *61*, 1307–1324.

Luce, Gay. *Body Time: Physiological Rhythms and Social Stress*. New York: Pantheon, 1971.

Luft, Joseph. *Of Human Interaction*. Palo Alto, Calif.: National Press, 1969.

Milio, Nancy. Dimensions of consumer participation and national health legislation. *American Journal of Public Health*, 1974, *64*, 357–363.

Paul, Benjamin (Ed.). *Health, Culture and Community: Case Studies of Public Reactions to Health Programs*. New York: Russell Sage, 1955.

Proshansky, Harold, Ittelson, William, & Rivlin, Leanne (Eds.). *Environmental Psychology: Man and His Physical Setting*. New York: Holt, Rinehart and Winston, 1970.

Public Law 93-641, Washington, D.C., U.S. Government Printing Office, 1975.

Reich, Wilhelm. *Wilhelm Reich: Selected Writings: An Introduction to Orgonomy*. London: Vision Press, 1973.

Schoen, Elin & Halprin, Lawrence. Humanizing the city environment. *The American Way*, November, 1972, pp. 12–23.

Smith, Alfred (Ed.). *Communication and Culture: Readings in the Codes of Human Interaction*. New York: Holt, Rinehart an Winston, 1966.

Soleri, Paolo. *Archology: The City in the Image of Man*. Cambridge, Mass.: MIT, 1969.

Soleri, Paolo. *The Bridge Between Matter and Spirit: Is Matter Becoming Spirit: The Arcology of Paolo Soleri*. Garden City: Anchor, 1973.

Sparer, Gerald, Dines, George, & Smith, Daniel. Consumer participation in OEO assisted neighborhood health centers. *American Journal of Public Health*, 1970, *60*, 1091–1102.

Swanson, Bert. The politics of health. In Howard Freeman, Sol Levine, & Leo Reeder (Eds.), *Handbook of Medical Sociology*, Englewood Cliffs, N.J.: Prentice-Hall, 1972, pp. 435–455.

Vladeck, Bruce. Interest-group representation and the HSAs: health planning and political theory. *American Journal of Public Health*, 1977, *67*, 23–29.

4

CHAPTER FOUR

Elements of Pattern: The Distribution of Energy

Nodes, networks, and boundaries (or interfaces) provide the elements of a community's pattern of energy distribution. Pattern is a frozen section of organization. It is a static description of structure. Organization provides the moving, dynamic description of its function.

Nodes, Networks, and Boundaries

Health

The distribution of energy is a function of the combined elements of nodes, networks, and boundaries. Health is dependent upon both the adequate distribution of energies to support growth, and the adequate constraint of the distribution of energies to maintain the pattern and uniqueness of the individual.

Community Health

The distribution of community energies is a function of the combined elements of nodes, networks, and boundaries.

These elements of a community's pattern (Doxiades, 1970; Lynch, 1960) may be applied to both weighted and unweighted energies. These elements are:

Nodes, central sources of community energies, may be centers of either weighted or unweighted energies. The most visible nodes of community energies are often found at the centers of transportation networks. Many cities grew up in response to crossings of different types of transportation systems. New York City grew at the point where water transport switched to land transport. Other cities grew at the point where canals met road or rail transport. Many forms of energy travel along transportation networks and gather at their centers. Barter or economic energies, material products, information, and caring or helping energies all tend to flow along transportation networks to various degrees and to gather at the centers. The centers which form at such crossings are often the most visible nodes of the community, and provide a place where we can begin to identify energy nodes within the community.

Networks carry both weighted and unweighted energies. Unweighted energy such as information flows through networks (Singh & Pareek, 1969). The "grapevine" is essentially an information network somewhat like the central nervous system of a community. New York's subway and London's underground system are weighted, transportation networks. The network which existed in the "underground" of the Second World War carried unweighted information and provided energies for action.

Boundaries to the distribution of energy exist as either weighted or unweighted energy forms in themselves. Space and time may also function as boundaries to the distribution of energy. Boundaries may be visible in themselves—such as a high wall that keeps prisoners in jail (Sommer, 1974); or by their effects—the backlog of energies which develops behind them. The long line waiting to get past the clinic clerk provides an example of this. Boundaries in living systems function as interfaces and are considered in this capacity in figures 27–30.

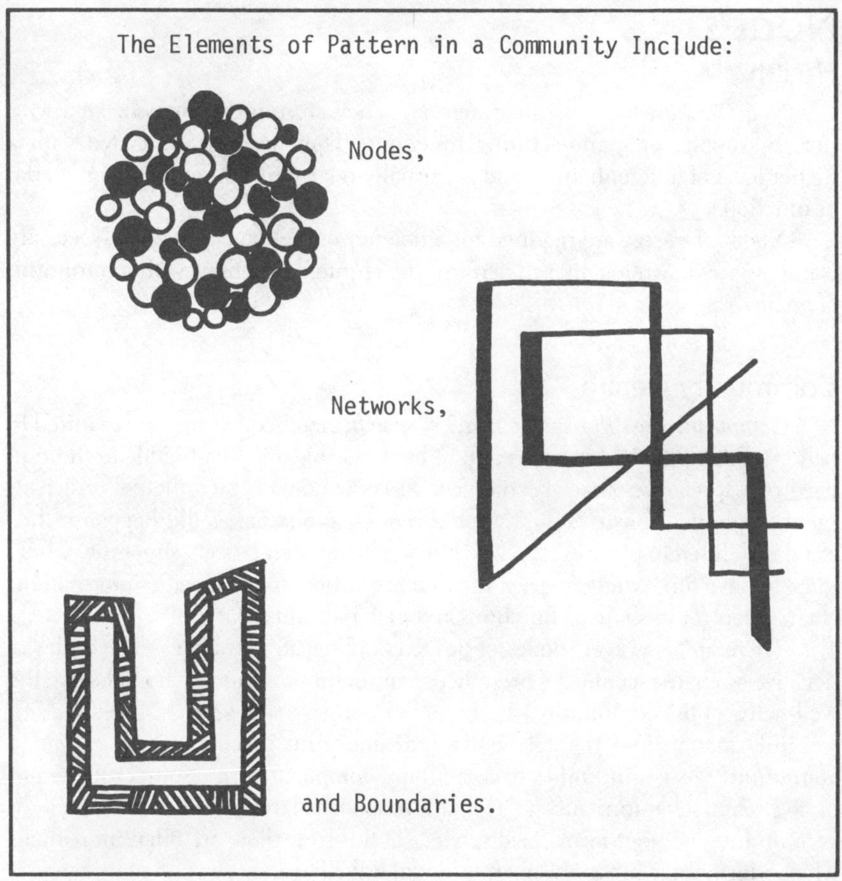

The Elements of Pattern in a Community Include:
Nodes,
Networks,
and Boundaries.

Community Health Assessment

What are the major nodes, or areas of concentrated energy? Where is the highest concentration of people? Where is the highest concentration of people with the greatest needs? Where do most of the families with young children live? Where do most of the older people live? Where are the recreation nodes, the healing nodes?

Where are the networks for transportation (roads, bus and subway lines), for information (who talks to who), for caring?

What are the major boundaries? Where are the "tracks" in your town? Who lives on the other side? What is, in fact, the boundary—a road, a river, or the proverbial railroad track itself? Are there political boundaries, such as zoning laws? Are there attitudinal boundaries, such as racial or economic prejudice, or both?

Nodes

Health

Nodes are areas of increased density. They are most often associated with storage, supply, or manufacturing functions. They are also associated with a higher level of differentiation, and are usually related to a differentiated material or function.

Nodes of energy are required for efficiency of the total organism. Necessary elements are drawn together to perform the required functions with a minimum of energy.

Community Health

Community health requires nodes of specific resources. Nodes are required to perform differentiated functions and to be accessible and identifiable to those in need of a specific resource. People need to know how to reach the police department by phone, how to get to the emergency room (what would happen if they put it in a different place every week?), where to do their grocery shopping, where to go to have fun, where to get some exercise, where to get specific information, etc. Centers for specialized functions and materials must exist.

There are, however, nodes of positive and negative energies. The nodes of negative energies—centers of prejudice, fear, dehumanization—do not serve the well-being of the community.

Information and referral centers are one form of energy node within a community. As communities become more complex, these resources move out of the realm of informality to formally established nodes (Dalton, 1952). In communities without formalized services of this sort, there are often individuals who perform these functions in an informal way. The lady down the block who is a nurse, the family doctor who is also a friend, the pharmacist who takes the time to chat, all are informal information and referral nodes within a community.

Nodes of ethnic culture in an area are often visible from the names of small stores. Recreational nodes are usually visible from the amount and quality of space they require. Educational nodes carry their own styles and sizes of buildings, and are surrounded by swarms of children at the beginning and end of the school day.

Other, less formal, nodes are more difficult to identify. The individual or group who will respond to a need of a specific group within the community is often difficult to identify. Telephone books provide access to information about formalized agencies and services. Only the grapevine provides access to information about informal agents and services. Those who have been in the community for a long time and those with specialized services to perform within the community are those most likely to know the informal nodes of specific resources.

On the other hand, nodes may be the result of a backup of energies behind some barrier, and result from the inability of a weighted or unweighted energy to

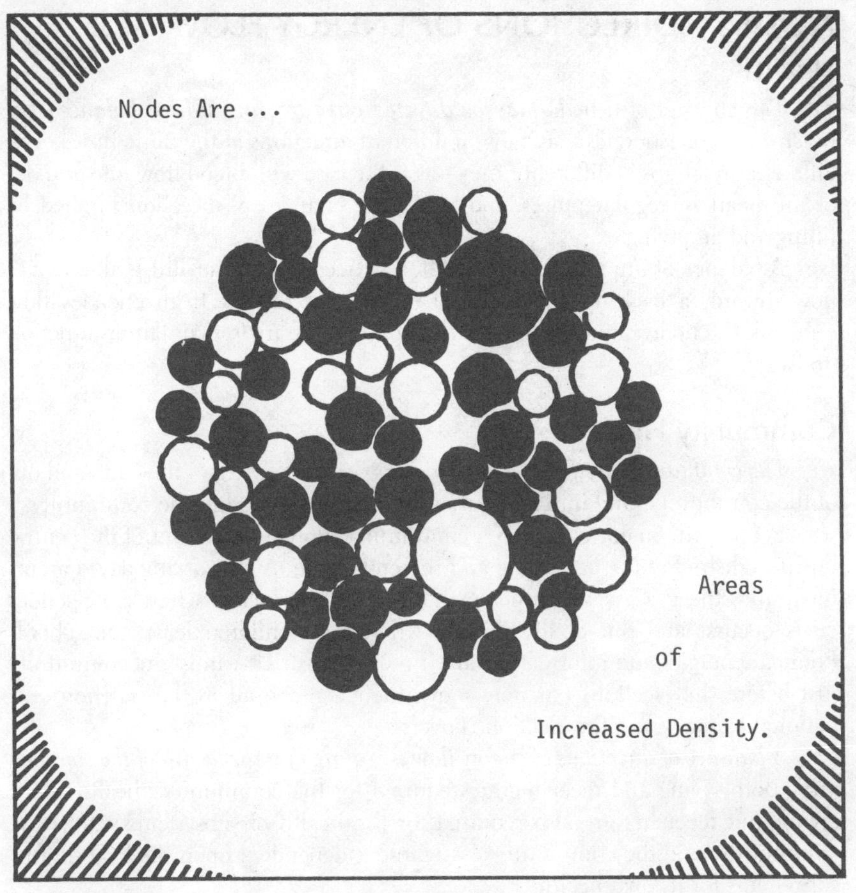
Nodes Are ...
Areas
of
Increased Density.

cross over a barrier. The psychological notion of repression is an example of this phenomenon.

Community Health Assessment

Identify the nodes for the relevant need and the relevant resource. Where are the people with the greatest need? Where is the highest concentration of people with the resource to meet that need?

Often, in community health, one is most interested in an unweighted energy source, and an informal resource to meet the need. Access to information in these areas can often be found from people who are in a related formal service, and who carry similar values and attitudes about the need in question. For example, a member of the La Leche League, holding strong values about caring in the mothering process, may know those in the community who are involved in planning new parent support groups.

NODES – DIRECTIONS OF ENERGY FLOW

Health

The energies of a node may be directed outward, inward, or balanced between the two. Energies may flow in different directions at the same time, or in different directions at different times—as is the case with blood flow into and out of the heart in regular pulses, indicating the changes of direction implied by filling and emptying.

A balance of inward and outward flow is necessary for health. If all energies flow inward, a back up and overload of energies results. If all energies flow outward, the node cannot maintain the supply necessary to maintain its function (to live).

Community Health

The community itself is a node, an energy center. Energies flow into and out of the community, and into and out of different nodes within the community.

People, the major energy of a community, flow into and out of the central business district at the beginning and the end of the usual working day. Parents move into the P.T.A. when their children enter school, or when some school crisis occurs, and out of the P.T.A. when their children leave the school. Political energies and information may flow into districts within the community just before the election, but may move their centers out to the statehouse or national capital when the election is over.

A *balance of directions of energy flow is required for the health of the community.* Both giving and receiving are required for the community's health. Both giving and receiving are also required for the health of subsystems within the community, and the community as a whole is dependent upon the health of its subsystems for its own health.

In the "good old days," when the family doctor was the total source of healing energies within the community, and constant demands were placed on his services, he was likely to burn out. Often, those most able to be altruistic maintain their energy with independent sources for caring input.

Many of the formal "helping" institutions in communities, whose stated goals and objectives are most idealistic, have turned their focus to the less formal goals of surviving as the sources of energy they need to maintain their functions become scare. Hospitals, educational institutions, and even community nursing agencies can no longer move outward to meet the needs of the community as completely as they once did. Rather, they must focus some of their energies on finding methods to draw energies inward to meet their own severe economic needs.

Community Health Assessment

What level of energy flows in and out of the community as a whole, and through the various nodes within the community? What is the balance of energy flow throughout the community?

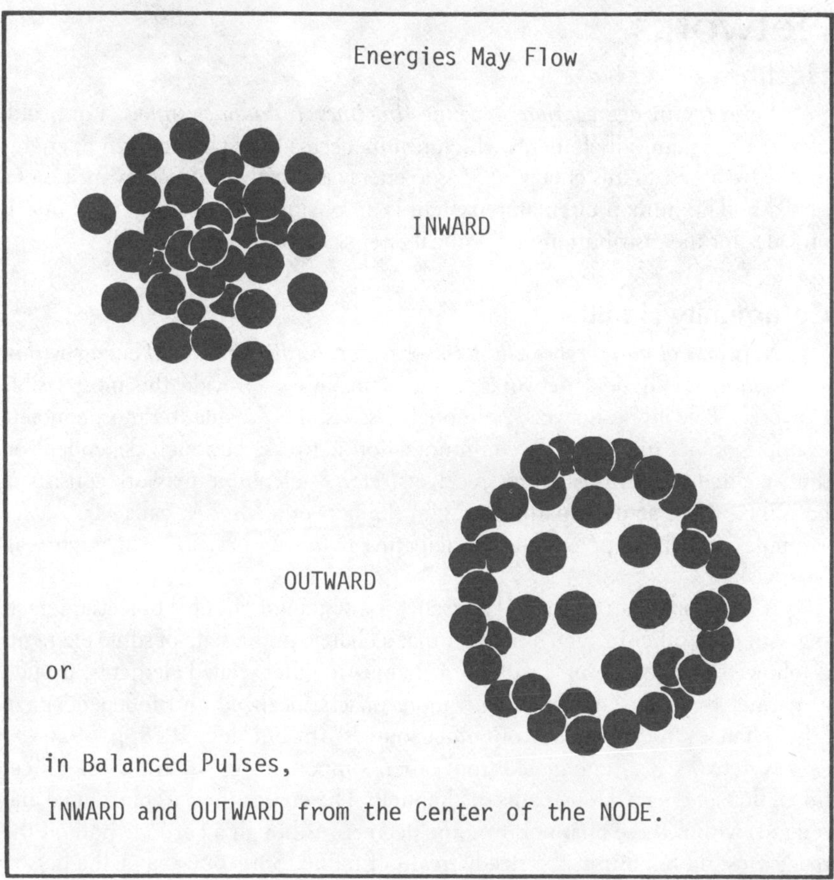

Energies May Flow
INWARD
OUTWARD
or
in Balanced Pulses,
INWARD and OUTWARD from the Center of the NODE.

Where do the nodes that appear to be constantly "giving" receive the resources necessary to maintain their function and to grow? What energies flow into these nodes to maintain their vitality? What types of nodes gather all energies toward their centers and what are the backlogs which result from this? Withholding information essential for intelligent planning is a frequent political strategy. Does this occur, and if so, at what price to the community? How does the local health planning agency disseminate information to the community? What human, informational, attitudinal, and economic energies does it draw to itself?

Networks

Health

Networks are aggregations of connecting lines, links, or channels. For health of a living system, all elements which *require* access to a specific form of energy must *have* access to this energy. Access to energy is usually provided by means of a network. The human circulatory system is an obvious example of a network. It provides for the distribution of chemical energies throughout the body.

Community Health

Networks of many types and forms exist for the distribution of energy within a community. Physical networks, such as roadways, provide the most visible networks. Telephone networks, although less visible, provide the most concrete example of an "unweighted" communication network, although dependent on the weighted elements of wires, receivers, etc. A telephone network consists of both the people actually participating in the network (Mrs. A. calls Mr. B., for example) and those potentially participating (Mrs. A. has not, but might call Mrs. C.).

A "network," according to Deutsch, "is a system of physical objects interacting with each other in such a manner that a change in the state of some elements is followed by a determinate pattern of changes in other related elements, in such a manner that the changes remain more or less localized and independent of other changes in the system from other sources" (in Buckley, 1968, p. 392).

A network is differentiated from other components of pattern by the directional flow of energy along paths or channels. The energy flow is constrained and remains within these channels to some degree. (Although a car may pull off the road, most do remain in the steady tream of traffic. Someone may tell a person outside the grapevine the latest gossip, but most of the news travels along the usual grapevine, and is not told to outsiders).

Community networks are the underpinnings of its health. The level of development of networks which carry differentiated types of energy reflect the level of development of the community. Well-differentiated networks with specific functions reflect the level of differentiation of that energy in a specific community. For example, in a commune, the level of differentiation regarding alternate modes of healing may be very high. An underground network for disseminating this information may also exist between several communes in the area. Information regarding informal sources of, and methods for, care would move along this network rapidly and efficiently. In a suburban neighborhood, there is more likely to be a high level of differentiation of information regarding formal sources of medical care. Information about a specific pediatrician in reference to a child's need would move through the latter network rapidly and efficiently. Information about an alternate method of healing would not move through the suburban network regarding formal methods of care as rapidly.

In some organizations, there may be a great deal of pressure to keep certain types of information restricted to certain members of the organization in order to

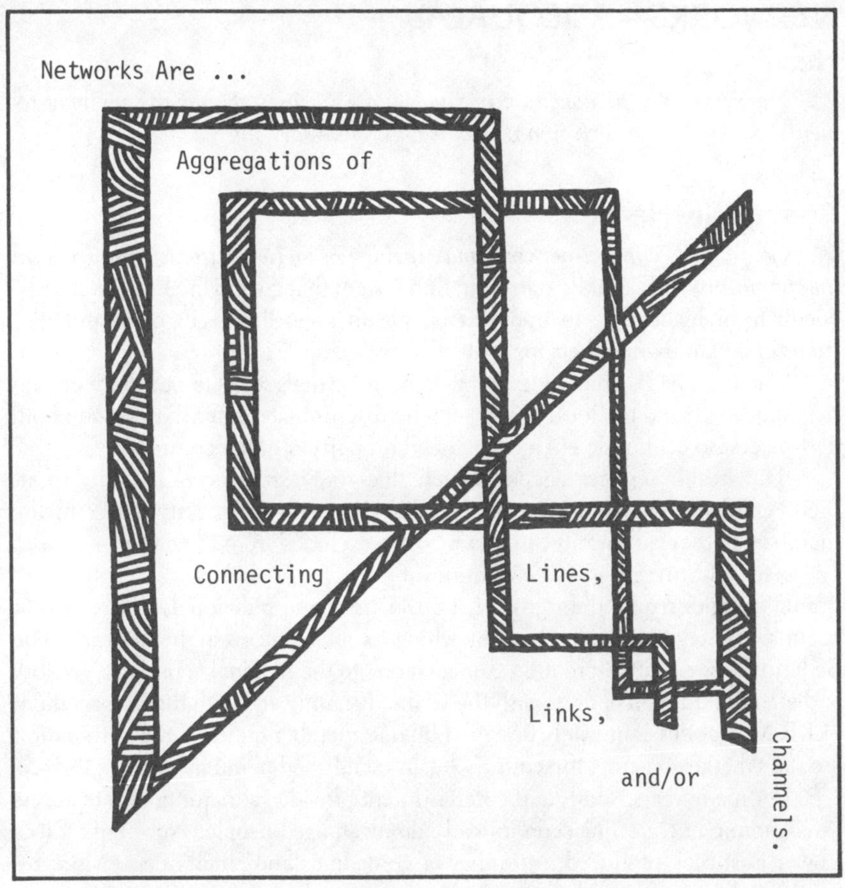
Networks Are ...
Aggregations of
Connecting
Lines,
Links,
and/or
Channels.

facilitate the maintenance of control by those in power. Extra effort may have to be expended to gain and maintain access to information in this situation. One nurse in a hospital setting made regular "rumor rounds" in order to have access to the information she needed to do her job (Savely, 1976).

Community Health Assessment

What are the major material "weighted" networks in the community? What necessary elements of the community are in contact with those networks? Which are not? Does the bus go to the hospital? Does it go to the low-cost grocery chain (Jakob, 1971)?

What would you expect the major informal networks to be? How would you gain access to them? Who might be in contact with the network about alternate forms of healing, about prenatal care, or about latest methods in child-rearing techniques? Is there a network of people interested in the socially isolated, in those out of contact with any human network?

NETWORKS—ADEQUACY

Health

Networks may be adequate or inadequate to meet the organism's requirements, depending on inclusion or exclusion of necessary subsystems.

Community Health

Community support networks may include or exclude various groups within the community. The public transportation system that goes to the hospital may be adequate or inadequate to transport people to meet the needs of hospitalized friends and family members for visits. (Markovitz, 1971).

The local bank which does not give homeowner's loans to people in certain neighborhoods and the local employer who discriminates against any group both deny access to economic energies to a certain portion of the community.

The health services agency which does not assure accountability of its members denies access to the decision-making network and its power to the members of the community at large who are excluded from the group.

Bedford-Stuyvesant was a community which had little access to the economic energies required for growth. Foundations and individuals with access to economic energies provided links by which to obtain access to the network. The Bedford-Stuyvesant Corporation gained access to the national economic network and energies through contact with the Kennedy family and with the management of I.B.M. Fabrics exquisitely designed by one member group of the corporation are now marketed across the country by an established manufacturer.

For many years, sports and entertainment provided a major means of access to economic energies for economically disadvantaged people. New York City's Lower East Side produced a number of comedians and entertainers. More recently, political and legislative action has attempted to open access to education and employment, as major links to economic networks and energies.

Inclusion or exclusion of individuals and groups from the networks of the community affects the health of the individual groups and the community itself. The socially isolated members of the community neither gain nourishment from the networks of the community, nor does the community gain from their potential contributions of sensitivity, information, or experience.

The deviants, the isolated, the neurotics, who choose not to be in contact with the usual community networks, miss a sense of relatedness, and the community loses the chance to hear the messages they present. (Goodman, 1955).

Drug pushers, gamblers, and prostitutes, form their own alternate networks and are excluded from the usual community business. State lotteries have attempted to bring gambling and gamblers into the "mainstream," but often with little success.

Alternate networks provide critical information for community health. They often anticipate more formal networks in responding to needs. They always provide messages about real community needs. The network of people in bars—

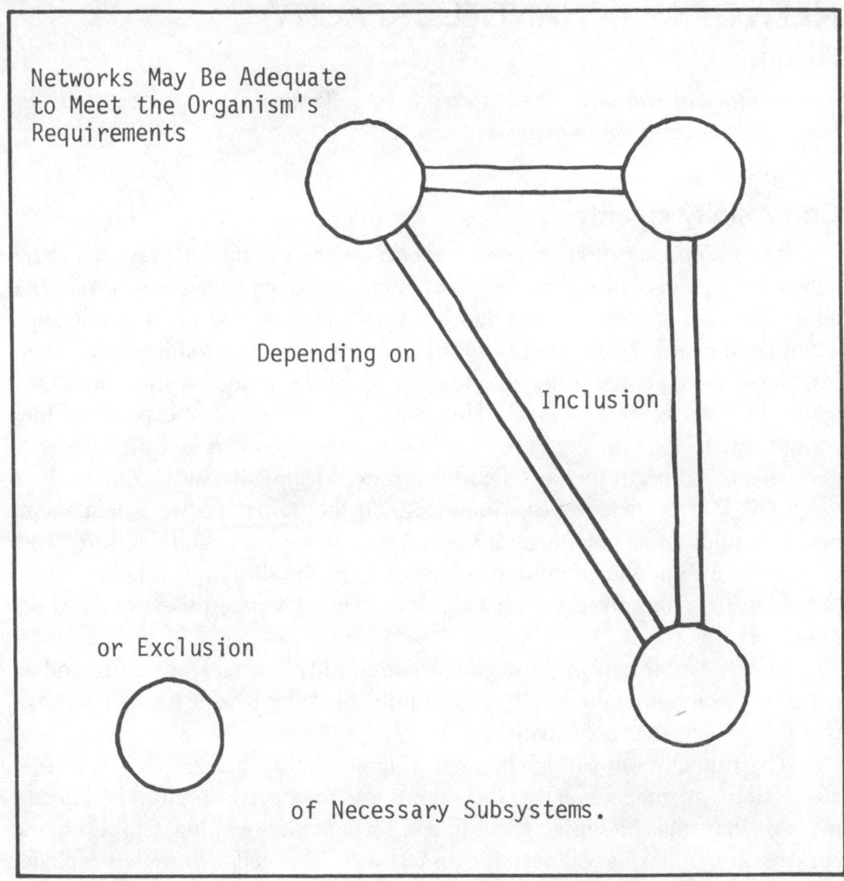
Networks May Be Adequate
to Meet the Organism's
Requirements
Depending on
Inclusion
or Exclusion
of Necessary Subsystems.

respectable bars or not-so-respectable bars—tell something about the community's lack of acceptance and lack of ability to meet their needs (Lyder, 1971).

Meals on Wheels programs bring the elderly isolated into contact not only with resources for good nutrition, but also with resources for socializing and give them a sense that somebody cares.

Community Health Assessment

If you are working in a community health agency, do you know what groups you do not reach? How many people are home alone, unable to get out, and without a telephone? What is the potential for developing some network to provide support and sharing for these people? Who gives support to the leaders of self-help groups?

NETWORKS – CHANNEL CAPACITY

Health

Insufficient channel capacities result in a backlog of unused energies and insufficient energies going to areas of need.

Community Health

Community networks are composed of channels and the links between channels. Channels may carry a greater or lesser amount of energy or may be selective about the types of energy which they can carry. The backlog which results from insufficient channel capacities is most clearly visible in the traffic jam analogy. Highways are supposed to be able to carry all of the traffic moving toward the center of the city at 8:45 A.M. However, in many people's experience they cannot. A backlog of energies occurs. People sit in their cars and their desire to get to work and begin the day often turns sour. Meanwhile, at the other side of the traffic jam, a trickle of cars moves out. If the traffic jam were permanent, people would not be able to get into town to do their work, and necessary work would remain undone. If no one arrived to open the shop, it would have to go out of business. If no trucks arrived to stock the grocery stores, they would go out of business.

In less visible terms, unweighted community energies of caring and of concern for other members of the community must also be able to move through invisible people-to-people channels.

The limitation of caring channels in large metropolitan areas is known to all. A smile at someone across the subway car may carry an entirely different message than that of simple friendly contact and well-wishing. However, the backlog of the unexpressed need for contact with one's fellow travellers explodes occasionally. The person with a puppy in a flight bag on a subway car may provide just the opportunity for the car full of strangers to smile and begin talking. The professional clown in the park reestablishes permission for contact between strangers.

The backlog of unused potential energy in the Mississippi Delta soil was released for the use of the hungry by the people of Mound Bayou.

A backlog of unexpressed feelings of the 1950's was released by the "soul" movement of the 1960's.

The backlog of potential energies for humanization of health care is just beginning to break through with programs built upon respect for the person being born (Leboyer, 1975) and for the person about to die (Kubler-Ross, 1975).

The health of communities depends upon channel capacities which are able to carry sufficient resources to all areas of need. Clear channels, open to give and to receive messages, are necessary. Prejudice and fear block the channels to expressions of warmth and human contact.

Fear of aging prevents communication with the elderly. Fear of emotions prevents communication with ethnic groups with greater skills in communication of feelings. Fear of loss of power prevents communication with those less

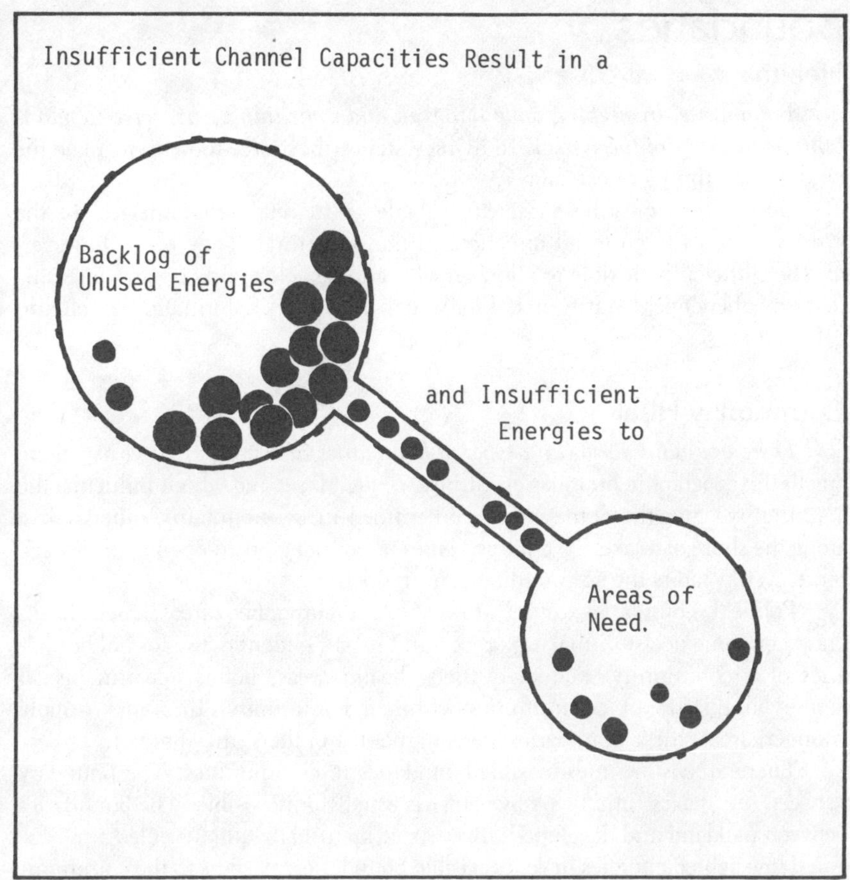
Insufficient Channel Capacities Result in a
Backlog of
Unused Energies
and Insufficient
Energies to
Areas of
Need.

privileged in the relevant area of power. Fear of perceiving prevents communication with the deviants of the community.

All of these limiting factors on the usual channels for communication prevent the objects of these fears from receiving the energies needed for their own growth. The elderly, the deviants of the community, and the isolated all require contact with the sources of information and caring and the sense of contact and identity which belonging to a community provides.

Community Health Assessment

Which channels in the community are sufficient, and which are insufficient, to carry energies of caring, concern, and relatedness? What channels in the community are able or unable to carry enough economic energies to meet the needs of specific community groups? What are the energies in the community that are most bottled up in certain areas? What are the areas which do not receive a sufficient supply of these energies?

Boundaries

Health

Boundaries, by keeping some things in and some things out, serve to maintain the integrity of the system. In living systems, they serve more to regulate the amount and timing of exchanges.

Boundaries must be sufficiently stable to maintain the integrity of the system—one can't go in all directions at the same time. They must, however, also be sufficiently flexible to allow growth, and be able to process an increasing diversity of energies (Maruyama, 1968), such as feelings, information, or chemical energies.

Community Health

There are many forms and types of boundaries in communities. First, there are all the geographic boundaries intrinsic to the place, and which influence the community's growth. Some cities are hemmed in by mountains, others curve along the shore of a lake. By contrast, cities unbounded on an open plain, spread more evenly across the surrounding countryside.

Political boundaries—cities, townships, incorporated areas, their limits drawn by some decision-making process in the past—identify the formal boundaries of a community. School districts, health areas, police departments all define boundaries of communities within a community. In some (usually younger) areas, these boundaries are congruent. In others, they are not.

There are visible and invisible boundaries in communities. The boundary between the "haves" and the "have nots" is usually quite visible. The boundaries between parkland and developed urban space are usually quite visible.

Unweighted energies have less visible boundaries. Barriers to the communication of caring or of anger exist in most communities. Personal walls against the perception of deviance exist. Faces turn away from the drunk on the stoop, as well as from the lovers who kiss on the street.

Culture provides barriers to some forms of self-expression while encouraging other forms. "All the news that's fit to print" provides a barrier to printing unfit news. "Family hour" provides a barrier to airing material deemed unfit for children to watch on television.

Time may present a barrier to certain resources or activities. A lifetime can only hold a certain number of accomplishments. An agenda may only allow for a limited number of issues.

Formal boundaries with incongruent lines for similar or overlapping information restrict ("bind") the information necessary to intelligent planning. The lack of relationship between significant bits of information is an additional barrier to the community's growth. For example, information about school achievement and child abuse may be significant data which would contribute to the community's ability to make an intelligent decision about funding for child abuse. If the board of education's and the police department's boundaries are not congruent, it may be more difficult to obtain this information.

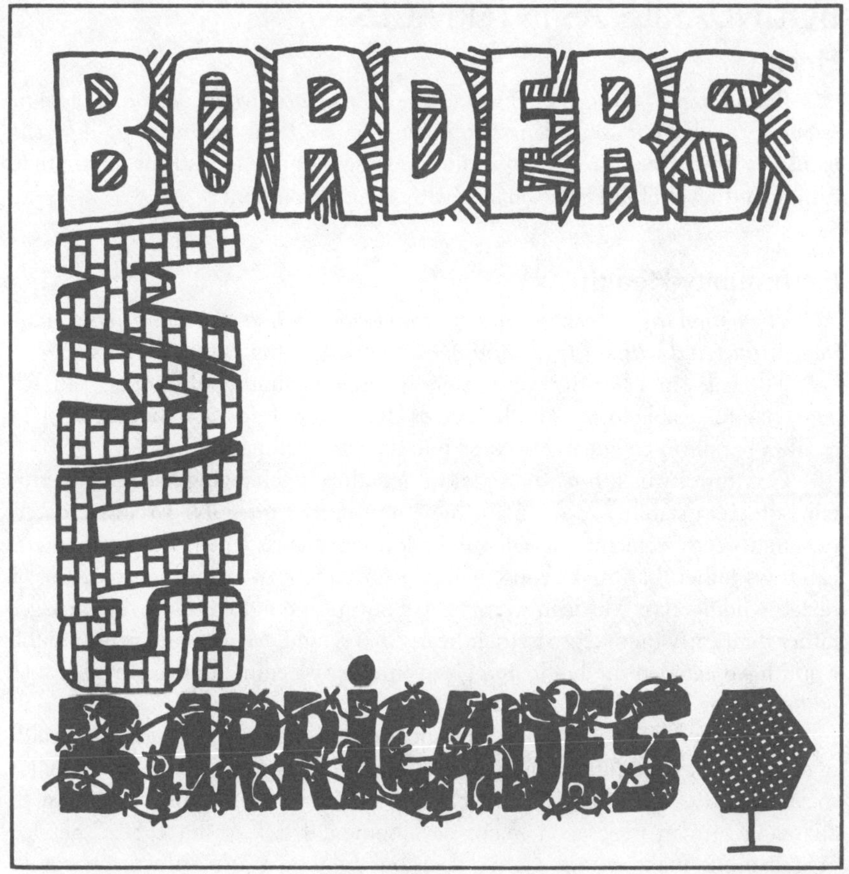

Informal boundaries may facilitate the community's order and integrity. Prohibitions against expressions of anger may reduce violence, and trauma, to others. On the other hand, they may also create fear of self-expression. Identifying and fostering the right balance is a challenge to early childhood teachers, responsible media decision makers, and nurses working with individuals and groups within the community.

Community Health Assessment

What are the formal boundaries of the community you have decided to study? What are the informal prohibitions and boundaries to self-expression? What negative elements are off-limits? Are they really negative? Are they negative for everyone? What positive energies are denied to what groups of people? What are the boundaries to the distribution of these energies—time, place, or administrative policies?

BOUNDARIES AS INTERFACES

Health

Boundaries in living systems function as interfaces which open and close in response to different conditions within and without the organism at different points in time. Health results from the increasing ability to find the appropriate timing and level of energy exchange with the environment.

Community Health

The boundaries in community open and close in response to different conditions within and without the organism at different points in time.

The gates to a healthy community in ancient times could not be "stuck." They had to be able to close in the face of attack, and they had to be able to open to allow people to go out and to come into the city at other times.

Community health requires that values adjust to changing needs, yet maintain sufficient stability to maintain the community's integrity. Excessive openness may occur in technologically underdeveloped areas which adopt all American ways rather than make conscious decisions about which values to accept or reject. Middle-class Mexican women may put their children in a baby carriage, rather than carry them close to their hearts in a serape. Many women around the world have adopted the bottle and given up breast feeding their infants because bottle feeding is the American way.

The flexibility of institutional boundaries is a major indicator of the health of communities. The inflexibility of institutional boundaries is one of the major social diseases of the late 1970's. Finding a way to loosen them to adjust to changing human needs is a major developmental task of the 1980's. Service organizations make administrative decisions to retract and reduce services in order to fulfill their own survival needs rather than the needs of their clients. More successful strategies for meeting client's needs should, however, result in higher revenues.

Computers establish barriers to communication of any information for which they are not programmed. Some of this blocked input would provide valuable information. Computers do facilitate the distribution of information. Barriers to the communication of personal data need to be maintained. Computers, as nonliving systems, do not respond to a changing balance of internal and external pressures. They respond to the input they were programmed to receive at some past point in time.

A tightly walled subsection of the community, bounded more by external than internal forces, may explode (as did Watts, and Harlem in the 1960's). Prisons, and mental institutions are similarly, tightly walled subsections of the community, with their primary walls built by external sources (Sommer, 1974).

Informal boundaries are often more flexible than formal boundaries. However, they may be less conscious, and more difficult to change due to the barrier of lack of awareness.

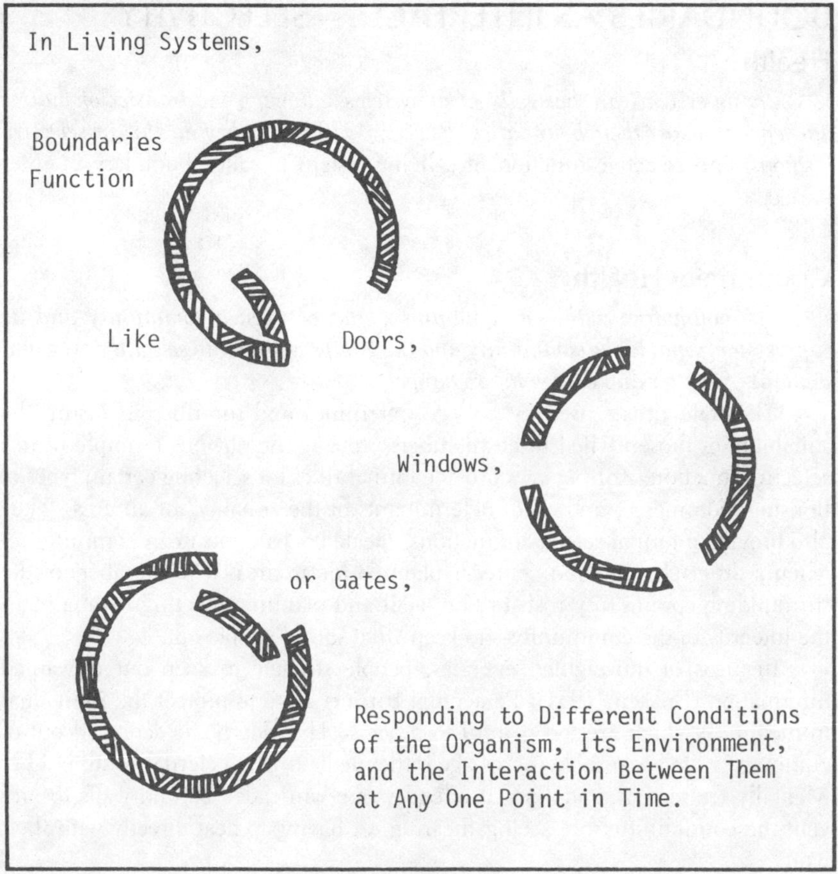

In Living Systems,
Boundaries
Function
Like
Doors,
Windows,
or Gates,
Responding to Different Conditions
of the Organism, Its Environment,
and the Interaction Between Them
at Any One Point in Time.

Community Health Assessment

What internal and external pressures are responsible for the most troublesome boundaries in your community? Which ones prevent the adequate distribution of health care? What internal and external pressures maintain them, what pressures serve to make them more flexible? What are the most troublesome boundaries to self-expression? What are the internal and external pressures that maintain them? What pressures produce change in the allowable types of self-expression?

What are the most effective boundaries to caring—between individuals, between groups? What internal and external pressures serve to open and close them? Simple lack of awareness can serve as a boundary. It can be one of the easiest boundaries to eliminate in a community.

BOUNDARIES AS INTERFACES—SELECTIVITY

Health

Living systems are basically open systems, allowing the transfer of matter and energy across their boundaries (Rogers, 1970), but they do this in selective fashion. This selective function of a living system is called boundary maintenance.

Community Health

The boundaries within a community, and between a community and its suprasystem, enable the community and the groups within it to select the type and amount of matter and energy for exchange.

Elaborate rituals used by college fraternities and sororities to insure the suitability of those invited to be members provide one obvious example of this selective function. Zoning laws provide formal rules for selecting certain types of housing, commerce, and other determinants of the "quality" of an area. They also provide informal selective functions. Heated debates occur in communities when a drug rehabilitation center is planned for an area. The members of the surrounding community rush to City Hall and planning meetings to maintain the integrity of the community—to keep "that sort of people out."

In areas of unweighted energies, people struggle to keep out unwanted information (Eriksen, 1951). Perceptual barriers serve to protect the individual from stimuli which are too painful to process. The elderly are screened out of community life because their message is the media myth of eternal youth is a lie. Mentally retarded and adolescent offenders are barricaded behind walls to prevent the community from seeing, hearing, or having to deal directly with their pain.

On the other hand, many communities expend a great deal of energy to recruit elements perceived as positive for the area. The chamber of commerce attempts to recruit new industry, new home buyers, additional tourists. Special programs attempt to draw new industry into the area. Club members and boards of nonprofit organizations may attempt to draw new members to their groups. Businesses attempt to bring in new customers.

The boundary maintenance functions of a community "select in" those elements necessary for it to maintain its functions and reject those elements which it perceives as negative. The selective function must be stable enough to allow for the continued integrity of the system, yet flexible enough to allow for its continuing growth. The organism must be able to become increasingly adept at its selection of elements for inclusion or exclusion of its definition of self.

Many communities provide evidence of their struggles in this area. Decisions to include or exclude a housing project, a different ethnic group, gay liberationists, or Gray Panthers become both more frequent and more conscious. The community struggles with its values to define and to accept or reject the proposals for a new building, a new program, or a new group of people.

The healthy community must be able to make effective decisions without

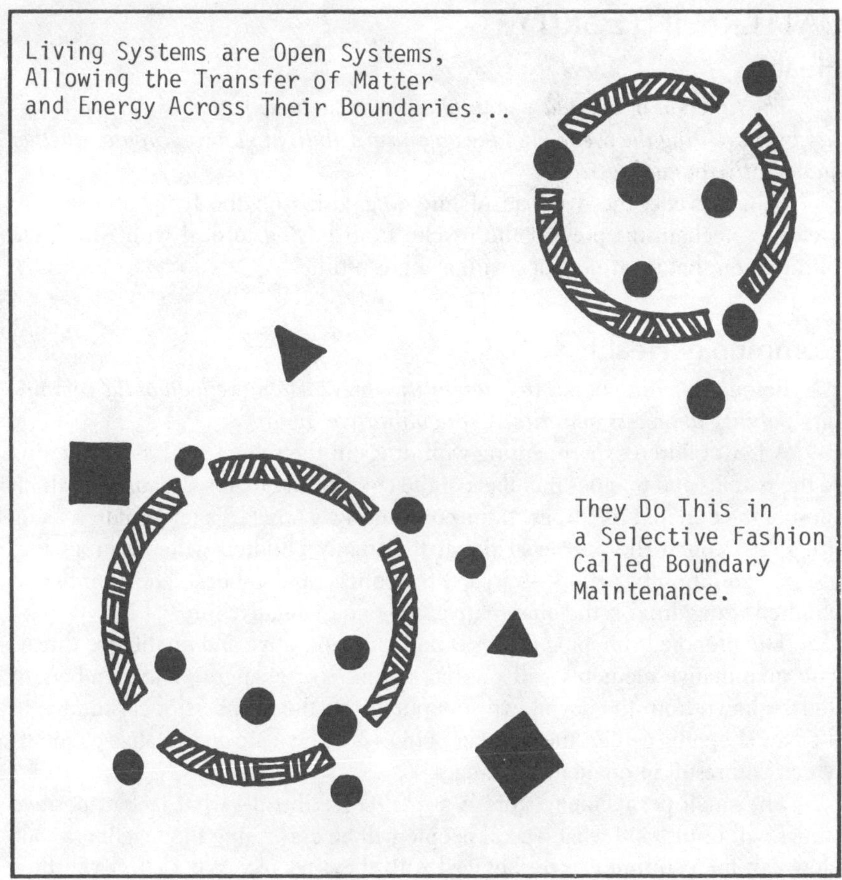
Living Systems are Open Systems,
Allowing the Transfer of Matter
and Energy Across Their Boundaries...
They Do This in
a Selective Fashion
Called Boundary
Maintenance.

denying either the rational or irrational needs of the members of the community.

The community's boundaries must be sufficiently efficient to prevent its loss of integrity. One cannot have the whole town demolished by a superhighway, a shopping center, or a new industry that brings in twice the current population of the town, and not loose the character of the people and the place.

Community Health Assessment

What weighted and unweighted elements does the community "select out"? Which ones does it seek to attract? What are the mechanisms by which this function occurs?

Who is excluded from participation in community decision-making groups? What elements are sought out for inclusion? Do the mechanisms by which the community seeks to maintain its integrity serve to reduce unwanted elements? Do they serve to attract and accept wanted elements? Are these mechanisms sufficiently flexible to allow community growth? Are they sufficiently stable to maintain its integrity?

PATTERN INTEGRITY

Health

The function of boundary maintenance is the preservation of pattern integrity by preventing the overload of the organism's ability to process inputs, whether quantitative or qualitative.

Skin prevents the overload of microorganisms on the lymphatic system. Defense mechanisms prevent the psyche from having to deal with issues and information that it cannot cope with at a given time.

Community Health

Boundary maintenance in communities prevents an overload of the community's ability to process quantitative or qualitative inputs.

A few children experimenting with drugs in the school are less threatening to the parents and to other members of the community than a situation in which most of the children use drugs. If the community is upset by a few children using drugs, it is often the perceived threat that many children will use drugs that arouses community action—by parents, police, and others. The number of children using drugs is the quantitative side of a qualitative threat.

The proposed shopping center is both a quantitative and qualitative threat. The quantitative elements will produce qualitative changes. The numbers of dollars drawn from the downtown shopping area, the numbers of cars drawn to the new shopping center, the number of trees cut down are quantitative elements which will result in qualitative changes.

The small pornography store is a qualitative threat—what lack of positive values will result, and what type of people will be drawn into the neighborhood? How can the community possibly deal with these people? What effect will they have on the children?

Television produces both a quantitative and a qualitative threat. How much violence will be seen? How can the parents, teachers, and other members of the community deal with what that does to their children's values and perceptions about methods for solving interpersonal problems? Will the early childhood teachers be able to keep up with the children's head start from educational television programs (Murray, Rubinstein & Comstock, 1972)?

Sanitation laws prevent the community from having to deal with an overload of disease producing micro-organisms. Values and mores prevent the community from having to deal with an overload of destructive behavior.

Community development plans prevent the community from having to deal with a sudden, unplanned influx of children into the school system.

Efforts to remove people from mental hospitals and place them back in the community are met with resistance, especially in communities where the population is unskilled and unsophisticated in dealing with mental illness. Strategies for community health would include assisting the community to increase its ability to deal with mental illness and deviant behavior before asking it to be able to accept an influx of people with these problems.

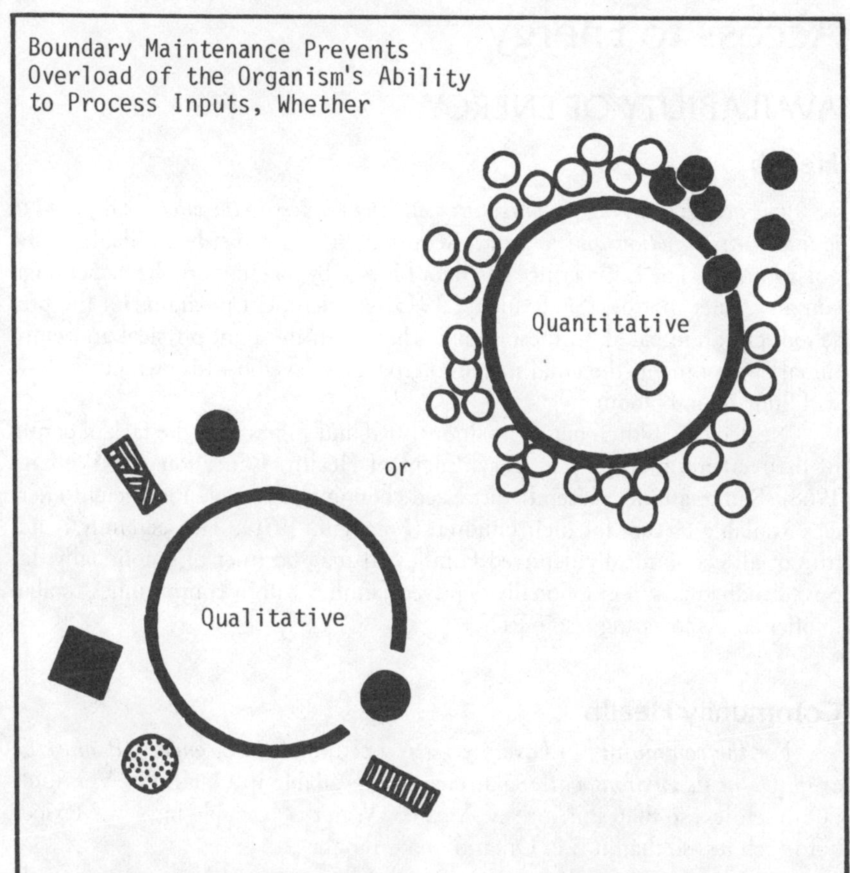
Boundary Maintenance Prevents
Overload of the Organism's Ability
to Process Inputs, Whether
Quantitative
or
Qualitative

Community Health Assessment

What are the perceived threats in the community? Are they quantitative, qualitative, or both? Is it a matter that the community can learn to cope with, or one that really overloads its ability to maintain its character and cope with the necessities of daily life?

Access to Energy

AVAILABILITY OF ENERGY

Health

The health of an organism requires sufficient access to the energies required to maintain its function and to grow. Required energies must be available in the environment. The Little Prince cared for his rose by making sure she had enough sun and water to grow (St. Exupery, 1945). Enrichment programs for the preschool child are based on the principle that given the right physical and emotional environment, the child's need to grow and develop—his own curiosity—will flourish and bloom.

Neglected children appear malnourished and suffer from the lack of caring in their environment (U. S. Department of Health, Education and Welfare, 1968). Some families, severely distressed economically, have insufficient energies available to care for their children (Freeman, 1970). This certainly is not true of all economically deprived families. It may be truer of emotionally deprived individuals in emotionally deprived families within communities unable to offer access to caring resources.

Community Health

For the community to have access to a certain form of energy, it must be available in its environment. Solar energy is available in Ontario or Vermont, but much less so than it is in New Mexico. Water is available in New Mexico, but much less so than it is in Ontario or Vermont.

Access to economic energies requires that there be economic energies available in the environment. You cannot squeeze water from a rock, as the old saying goes. Low income groups who have gained economic power have done so by directing their activities to sources of economic power. The entertainment industry is directed at those with dollars over and above the requirement for survival. You would never get rich entertaining people with severe economic needs. It may well be that there will never be a redistribution of physicians to rural areas until there are unemployed physicians in developed areas. Nutrition programs for the poor depend on a sufficient supply of food for everyone. Should a famine occur, food stamps and programs for malnourished mothers and infants will fall into disfavor. Many of the liberals of the sixties have become more conservative as the tax bite of the seventies hits their purses.

A community requires access to energies within its environment in order to maintain its function and to achieve its next level of development.

Weighted environmental resources, breathable air, drinkable water, safe recreation spaces now require planning for their continued accessibility as the threats of scarcity increase.

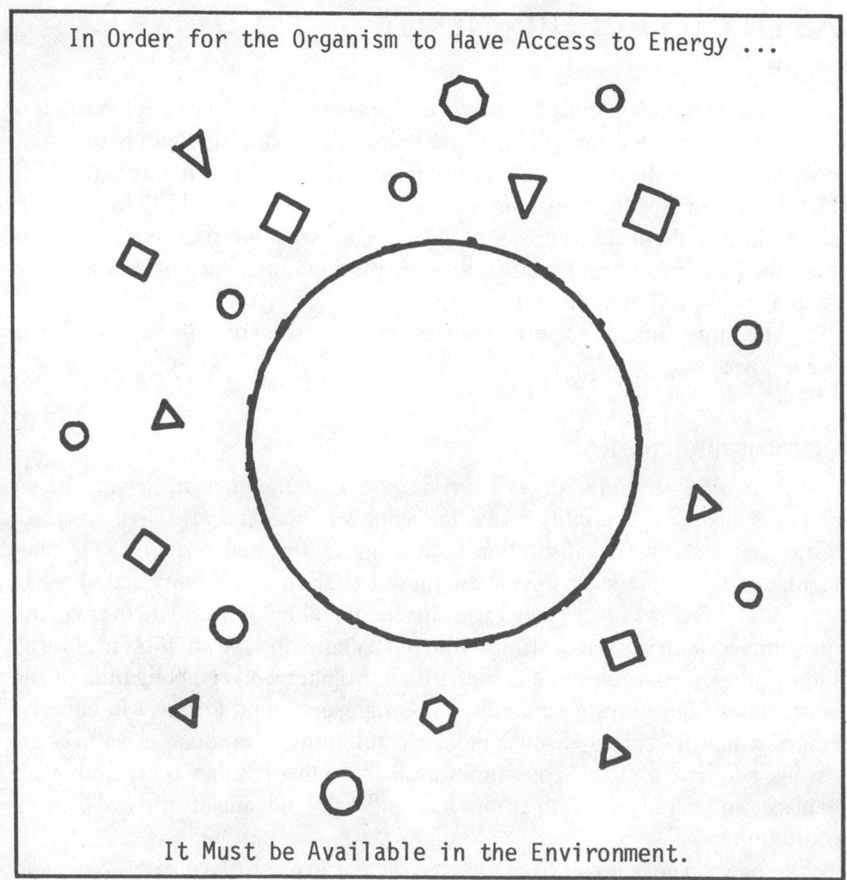
In Order for the Organism to Have Access to Energy ...
It Must be Available in the Environment.

Unweighted environmental resources, hope, caring, and values such as honesty are more available in some environments than in others.

Hope, a real form of unweighted energy, may be lacking in the community or in its environment.

The need for more humanistic approaches to the birth process was felt by many men and women. However, until information about an alternate method, *Birth Without Violence* (Leboyer, 1975), was available in the environment, there was no way for most people to take effective action to meet that need.

Community Health Assessment

What necessary energies are available in the community's environment? What energies are not available in your community's environment? What energies are scarce and require planning to maintain their continued existence in the environment?

ABILITY TO ACCEPT ENERGY

Health

Any living system must be open to accept energies which are available to it in its environment. Once accepted, it must also be able to assimilate them into its own pattern. Malnutrition can result from lack of access to nutrients (U.S. Department of Health, Education & Welfare, 1968, pp. 117–119); from lack of ability to take them into the system (as in esophageal atresia, for example); or from the inability to digest or assimilate the nutrients once they have entered the system (as in PKU or cystic fibrosis).

The same principles apply to inadequate nourishment with regard to learning or love.

Community Health

A *community may be malnourished from its inability to accept outside resources or from its inability to use the resources once they have been accepted.* (One large state mental institution built a marvellous new building. The state legislature then refused to provide the funds to staff it, and it remained unused.)

"Culture shock" is the label used for the inability to assimilate overwhelming numbers of new ideas or stimuli into old patterns and the attempts to close off some of the excessive stimuli (Toffler, 1970). Migrant workers, both affluent and poor, suffer from excessive mobility, although some tend to travel in cohesive groups which provide their own mobile community. Corporate executives are less likely to have a mobile community available to them as they move from place to place, and job to job. Both groups have difficulty in being assimilated by local communities.

In order to have access to energy, the community must be able to accept and assimilate the energies available to it in its environment.

In ancient cities, no one could get water from a well outside the city gates if the gates were locked because the city was under attack. (Michener, 1965). The city was not open to seek or accept this resource. Even if the residents were able to plan a method to get the water through the gates, the city dwellers would have had to develop pottery jars or some other containers to store and distribute the water.

A more modern example of a community's lack of openness to an environmental resource is seen in some ethnic groups, which, in order to keep their women at home and under control, prohibit them from learning English. Another example is seen in the strong cultural conditioning of women to avoid men's jobs, thereby barring themselves from access to economic resources and professional satisfaction.

Community groups that seek to provide care for those members of the community who are in need can only be used as a resource if those in need are willing to accept their services. Many oriental groups hold strong cultural values against accepting help from outsiders. Often, an oriental nurse or other health

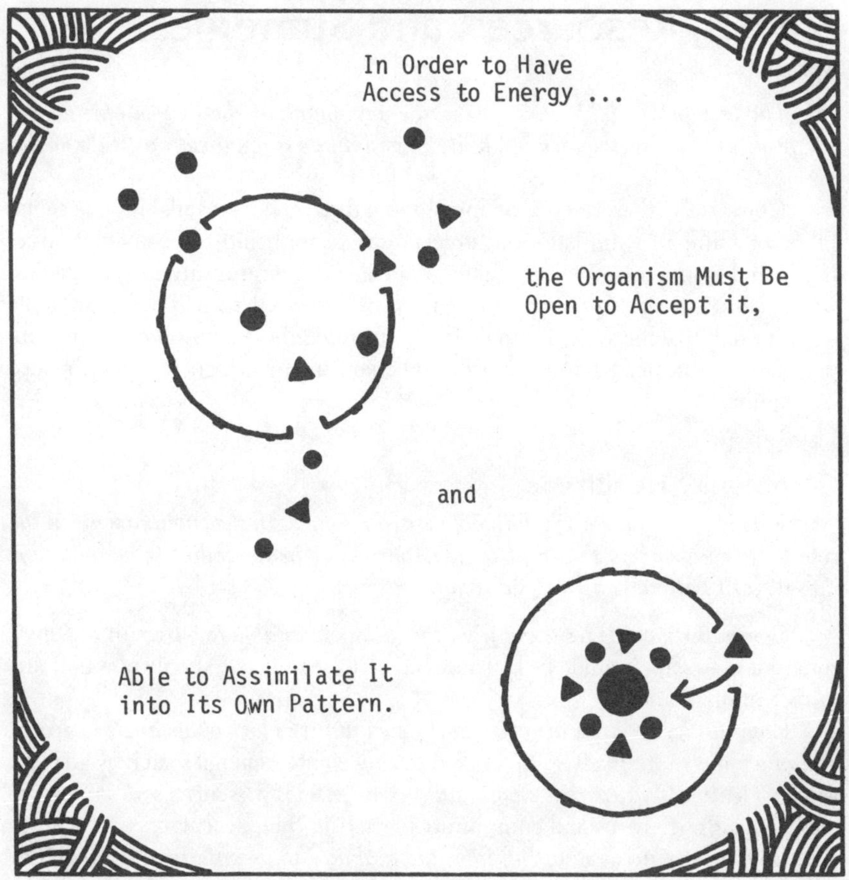
In Order to Have
Access to Energy ...
the Organism Must Be
Open to Accept it,
and
Able to Assimilate It
into Its Own Pattern.

care worker can bridge the gap which allows for the necessary openness to external resources.

Community Health Assessment

What resources which are available in the community's environment is it unable to accept, or to assimilate? Is the wisdom of older people unacceptable because of their age? Are changing attitudes in regard to violence on television capable of assimilation by sponsors and media decision makers?

Is the community able to accept some women's needs to work outside the home? Is it able to accept the needs of women who do choose to stay home with their children? Is the community able to provide understanding and resources such as day care centers to both groups of women? Is it able to assimilate both life styles into its own pattern of attitudes, values, and provision of services?

Needs, Resources, and Strategies

Health

The lack of available resources in the environment, the lack of openness to accept a resource, or the lack of ability to assimilate a resource constitute health needs.

Conversely, the presence of any of these three factors (availability, acceptability, or ability to assimilate) constitute a resource for health. Recombinations of needs and resources constitute major strategies for community health. Needs, when acute enough to provide some form of perceived pain, but not so acute so to immobilize the system, provide a stimulus to growth. Resources, when appropriate to the needs, constitute the mechanisms by which the growth need can be met.

Community Health

A *deficiency in the availability of desired resources in the environment, in the community's openness to accept these resources, or in its ability to assimilate it into its own pattern constitutes a community need.*

Community needs resulting from the lack of available resources in the environment may soon include lack of access to a sufficient, safe supply of water, air, or recreational land.

Community needs resulting from the community's lack of openness to accept a resource are more likely to be related to unweighted energies such as goals or values. *Health, Culture and Community* (Paul, 1955) presents a series of examples of health behaviors and community barriers to their acceptance.

Community needs resulting from the inability to assimilate a resource into its own pattern for processing energies can be seen in the struggles to achieve accountability in health care planning and delivery. Groups which were not previously used to having a say in the decision making process are challenged to do so. Groups which are not used to NOT having total control over their own practice are asked to share their decisions, and documentation of the care they give, with others.

Community health needs and resources can be identified on many levels. Overriding, acute needs for material resources are usually evident and visible at the first look. Community needs with regard to unweighted energies often require a great deal of time to uncover.

Community health results from the progressive perception and identification of needs, appropriate resources, and the successful resolution of each level of need.

A small subcommunity of mothers within a community may identify the need for a children's after-school program. They may identify those women in the group who are willing and able to watch a group of children once or twice a week, but not every day. They will then plan to meet this need, by using the

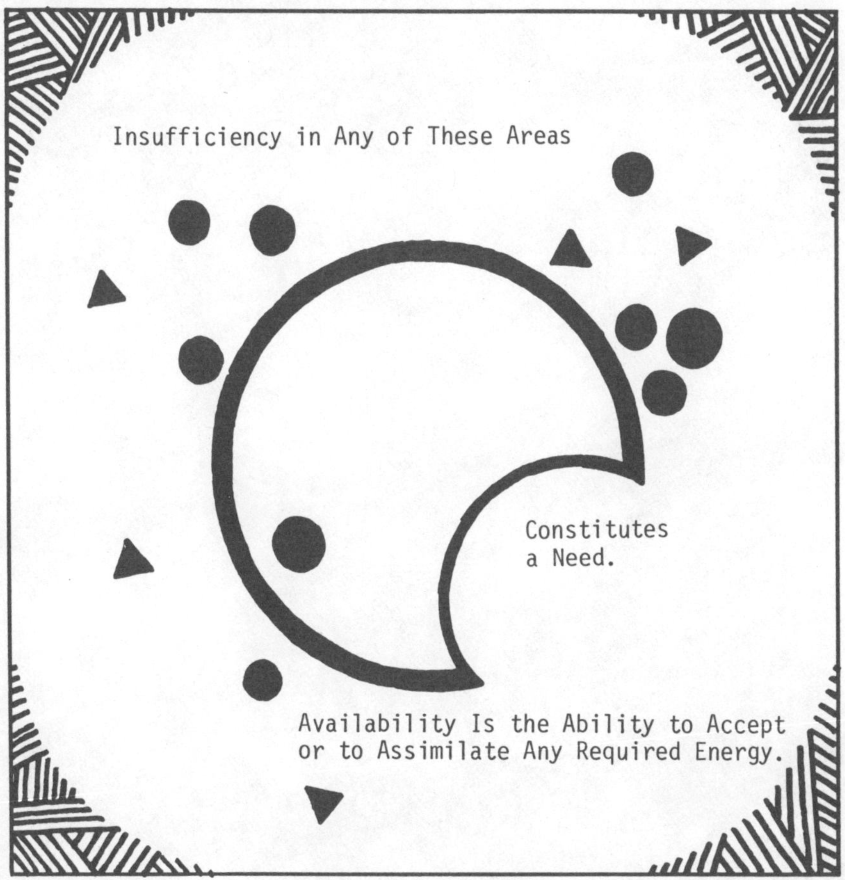

resources appropriately—one or two mothers a day, every day—and not 10 mothers on one day. The group identifies its need for space, and finds a resource for the space. After a time, the group may identify a need for assistance with behavioral problems of some of the children, and begin seeking a resource for such help. Increasingly sophisticated needs and their appropriate resources may be identified over time, as the center grows into a community resource in itself.

Insufficiency in Any of These Areas
Constitutes
a Need.
Availability Is the Ability to Accept
or to Assimilate Any Required Energy.

Community Health Assessment

What major health needs have you identified in your community? What major resources can you identify to meet these needs? What is the possibility of linking these needs with appropriate resources?

References and Resources

REFERENCES

Dalton, Melville. Formal and informal organization. In Amatai Etzioni (Ed.), *Readings on Modern Organizations*. Englewood Cliffs, N.J.: Prentice-Hall, 1969, pp. 114–121.

Deutsch, Karl. Toward a cybernetic model of man and society. In Walter Buckley (Ed.), *Modern Systems Research for the Behavioral Scientist: A Sourcebook*. Chicago: Aldine, 1968, pp. 387–400.

Doxiades, Constantinos. Ekistics, the science of human settlements. *Science*, 1970, **170**, 394–404.

Eriksen, C. W. Perceptual defense as a function of unacceptable needs. *Journal of Abnormal and Social Psychology*, 1951, *46*, 557–564.

Freeman, Ruth. *Community Health Nursing Practice*. Philadelphia: W. B. Saunders, 1970.

Gesell, Arnold, Ilg, Frances, & Ames, Louise. *Infant and Child in the Culture of Today*. (Revised Edition.) New York: Harper & Row, 1974.

Goodman, Paul. *Utopian Essays and Practical Proposals*. New York: Vintage, 1955.

Haddon, William. On the escape of tigers: an ecologic note. *American Journal of Public Health*, 1970, *60*, 2229–2234.

Jakob, Dorothea. Community health assessment: Mariners' Harbor. Unpublished paper, 1971.

Kubler-Ross, Elisabeth. *Death: The Final Stage of Growth*. Englewood Cliffs, N.J.: Prentice-Hall, 1975.

Leboyer, Frederick. *Birth Without Violence*. New York: Knopf, 1975.

Lyder, Roberta. Community health assessment. Unpublished paper, 1971.

Lynch, Kevin. *The Image of the City*. Cambridge, Mass.: MIT, 1960.

Markovitz, Joni. Transportation needs of the elderly. *Traffic Quarterly*, 1971, 25, 237–253.

Maruyama, Magoroh. The second cybernetics: deviation-amplifying mutual processes. In Walter Buckley (Ed.), *Modern Systems Research for the Behavioral Scientist: A Sourcebook*. Chicago: Aldine, 1968, pp. 304–313.

Michener, James. *The Source*. New York: Random House, 1965.

Murray, John, Rubinstein, Eli, & Comstock, George (Eds.). *Television And Social Behavior: Reports and Papers, Volume II: Television and Social Learning*. (A Technical Report to the Surgeon General's Scientific Advisory Committee on Television and Social Behavior, #1724-0195 Washington D.C.: U.S. Government Printing Office, 1972.

Paul, Benjamin. *Health, Culture and Community: Case Studies of Public Reactions to Health Programs*. New York: Russell Sage, 1955.

Rogers, Martha. *An Introduction to the Theoretical Basis of Nursing*. Philadelphia: F. A. Davis, 1970.

Ryan, William. *Blaming the Victim*. New York: Vintage, 1971.

Saint-Exupéry, Antoine de. *The Little Prince*. Harmondsworth, Middlesex, England: Penguin, 1945.

Saveley, Pam. Personal Communication. 1976.

Singh, Y. P., & Pareek, Udai. Communication nets in the sequential adoptation process. *Psychologia*, 1969, *12*, 232–246.

Sommer, Robert. *Tight Spaces: Hard Architecture and How to Humanize It*. Englewood Cliffs, N.J.: Prentice-Hall, 1974.

Toffler, Alvin. *Future Shock*. New York: Random House, 1970.

U.S. Department of Health, Education and Welfare; Public Health Service; National Institutes of Health; the National Institute of Child Health and Human Development. *Perspectives on Human Deprivation: Biological, Psychological and Sociological*. Washington, D.C.: U.S. Government Printing Office, 1968.

RESOURCES

Alexander, Christopher. *Notes on the Synthesis of Form*. Cambridge, Mass.: Harvard University, 1964.

Alinsky, Saul. *Reveille for Radicals*. New York: Vintage, 1969.

Arnstein, Sherry. A ladder of citizen participation. *Journal of the American Institute of Planners*, 1969, *35*, 216–224.

Bennis, Warren, Benne, Kenneth, & Chin, Robert (Eds.). *The Planning of Change*. New York: Holt, Rinehart & Winston, 1969.

Berrien, F. Kenneth. *General and Social Systems*. New Brunswick, N.J.: Rutgers University, 1968.

Buckley, Walter. *Sociology and Modern Systems Theory*. Englewood Cliffs, N.J.: Prentice-Hall, 1967.

Buckley, Walter (Ed.). *Modern Systems Research for the Behavioral Scientist: A Sourcebook*. Chicago: Aldine, 1968.

Carlson, Gail & Irene Ruys-Nelson. *The Discovery of Human Potentials*. Madison, Wisc.: Section of Child Behavior and Development, Bureau of Community Health Services, Division of Health, Department of Health and Social Services, 1971.

Chermayeff, Serge & Alexander, Christopher. *Community and Privacy*. Garden City: Anchor, 1965.

Chermayeff, Serge & Tzionis, Alexander. *Shape of Community: Realization of Human Potential*. Baltimore: Penguin, 1971.

Christakis, George (Ed.). Nutritional assessment in health programs. *American Journal of Public Health*, 1973, *63*. (Supplement to November, 1973 issue.)

Danaceau, Paul. *Consumer Participation in Health Care: How Its Working*. Arlington, Va.: Human Services Institute for Children and Families, 1975.

Flavier, Juan. *Doctors to the Barrios*. Quezon City, Phillipines: New Day, 1970.

Hall, Edward. *Beyond Culture*. Garden City: Anchor, 1977.

Halprin, Lawrence. *The RSVP Cycles: Creative Processes in the Human Environment*. New York: George Braziller, 1969.

Hill, Robert. *The Strengths of Black Families*. New York: Emerson Hall (Urban League), 1971.

Karagulla, Shafica. *Breakthrough to Creativity: Your Higher Sense Perception*. Marina Del Rey, Calif.: DeVorss, 1967.

Katz, D. & Kahn, R. L. *The Social Psychology of Organization*. (Second edition.) New York: John Wiley, 1978.

Latham, Michael & Francisco Cobos. The effects of malnutrition on intellectual development and learning. *American Journal of Public Health*, 1971, *61*, 1307–1324.

Lawrence, Paul & Lorsch, Jay. Differentiation and integration in complex organizations. In Joseph A. Litterer (Ed.). *Organizations: Systems, Control and Adaptation*. (Second Edition.) Vol. II. New York: John Wiley & Sons, 1969, pp. 229–253.

Leighton, Alexander, Mason, Edward, Kern, Joseph, & Leighton, Frederick. Moving Pictures as an Aid to Community Development. *Mental Health Digest*, 1972, 4, 1–5.

Lewin, Kurt. *Field Theory in Social Science: Selected Theoretical Papers*. New York: Harper, 1964.

Liston, Robert. *The American Poor: A Report on Poverty in the United States*. New York: Dell, 1970.

Milio, Nancy. *The Care of Health in Communities: Access for Outcasts*. New York: Macmillan, 1975.

Milio, Nancy. Dimensions of consumer participation and national health legislation. *American Journal of Public Health*, 1974, 64, 357–363.

Milio, Nancy. 9226 *Kercheval: The Storefront that Did Not Burn*. Ann Arbor: University of Michigan, 1970.

Miller, James. Living systems: basic concepts. *Behavioral Science*, 1965, **10**, 193–237.

Papenek, Victor. Designing environments for human potential. *Social Policy*, 1972, **2**, 24–29.

Redfield, Robert. Levels of integration in biological and social systems. In Walter Buckley (Ed.), *Modern Systems Research for the Behavioral Scientist. A Sourcebook*. Chicago: Aldine, 1968, pp. 59–68.

Shaw, Marvin, Rothschild, Gerald, & Strickland, John. Decision processes in communication nets. In Alfred Smith (Ed.), *Communication and Culture:*

Readings in the Codes of Human Interaction. New York: Holt, Rinehart and Winston, 1966, pp. 253–259.

Shapiro, Joan. Group work with urban rejects in a slum hotel. In William Schwartz & Serapio Zalba (Eds.), *The Practice of Group Work*. New York: Columbia University, 1971.

Spradley, James & Phillips, Mark. Culture and stress: a quantitative analysis. *American Anthropologist*, 1972, *74*, 518–529.

Suttles, Gerald. *The Social Order of the Slum: Ethnicity and Territory in the Inner City*. Chicago: University of Chicago, 1970.

Vladeck, Bruce. Interest-group representation and the HSA's: health planning and political theory. *American Journal of Public Health*, 1977, *67*, 23–29.

5

CHAPTER FIVE

Individuality: The Expression of Individual Goals

Individuality is the uniqueness of the individual—his gift to others and to himself of his spontaneous expressions of self.

Individuality is in itself a form of energy—the need to be creative, spontaneous, innovative. It is the expression of the human need for growth into being and becoming. It represents individual commitments and expressions of commitment. It is something which is unique and special to all living things, and most especially to human beings.

As a form of energy, individuality follows the same principles as other forms of energy. There are additional principles, however, which are particular to individuality. The directions which the energy provided by individuality take are tailored, in large part, by the goals and values of the person, group, or community.

Individuality represents the need for unplanned, here and now, authentic, spontaneous expressions of self: yes, no; love; caring; anger; joy; the pride of accomplishment; the sorrow of loss. These are the richest bits of the fabric of human life and expression.

Goals

Health

Goals, spoken or unspoken, aware or unaware, serve to organize the activities of the individual. Unspoken needs for survival, for interaction with others, for self-esteem and the esteem of others often go unnoticed. Unaware needs and goals, often expressed in spontaneous laughter, tears, or anger, speak of the unique qualities of the individual. Vacation plans and career plans are more conscious goals, and represent the need for the next level of development or for the access to resources to achieve this.

Community Health

The uniqueness of a community is rooted in central, organizing themes. Its goals, whether spoken or unspoken aware or unaware, provide these organizing themes. Communities of interest often have spoken, consciously arrived at, and stated goals (objectives) and purposes. Religious communities and educational and professional communities can most often state their goals. Communities which are bound to a place are less likely to be able to consciously state their overall goals. They may be able to state a specific goal in reference to a specific need. The planning commission may have established goals. Deeper goals, inherent in the community, lie in the deeper recesses of its collective consciousness, and may be more difficult to articulate. These less conscious goals are, no less, organizing themes which contribute to the uniqueness of the community.

Alexander, in his *Notes on the Synthesis of Form* (1964), presents the notion that goodness of fit often goes unnoticed. Rather, he says, it is the place where the shoe pinches that is felt. Therefore, it is the points of poor fit with the community's goals which provide the clues to the unspoken values and goals of the community. The reaction to a proposed shopping center in the middle of parkland; to the introduction of an off-colored book on the high school reading list; to a proposed superhighway—all provide clues to the community's goals. Preservation of contact with nature, preservation of traditional sexual mores, may be the goals underlying these areas of poor fit. On the other hand, when something of "good fit" is newly proposed or falls into place, it *is* recognized.

The notion of a critical mass—a group ready and waiting for the solution to a problem—which is large enough to produce effective action is useful in this area (Schlotfeldt, 1974). Oh yes, "why didn't we think of that before" is the response to an idea whose time has come, and which is consistent with the group's individual needs and goals. Ready acceptance of a bicycle lane, prohibitions against transport of nuclear wastes through the town, indicate communities which value physical activity and exercise, and wish to preserve an environment unaffected by technological spinoffs.

The goals in a community provide its central organizing themes. These central organizing themes are both expressions of, and a force which patterns further expressions of, the uniqueness of the community. Major goals, common

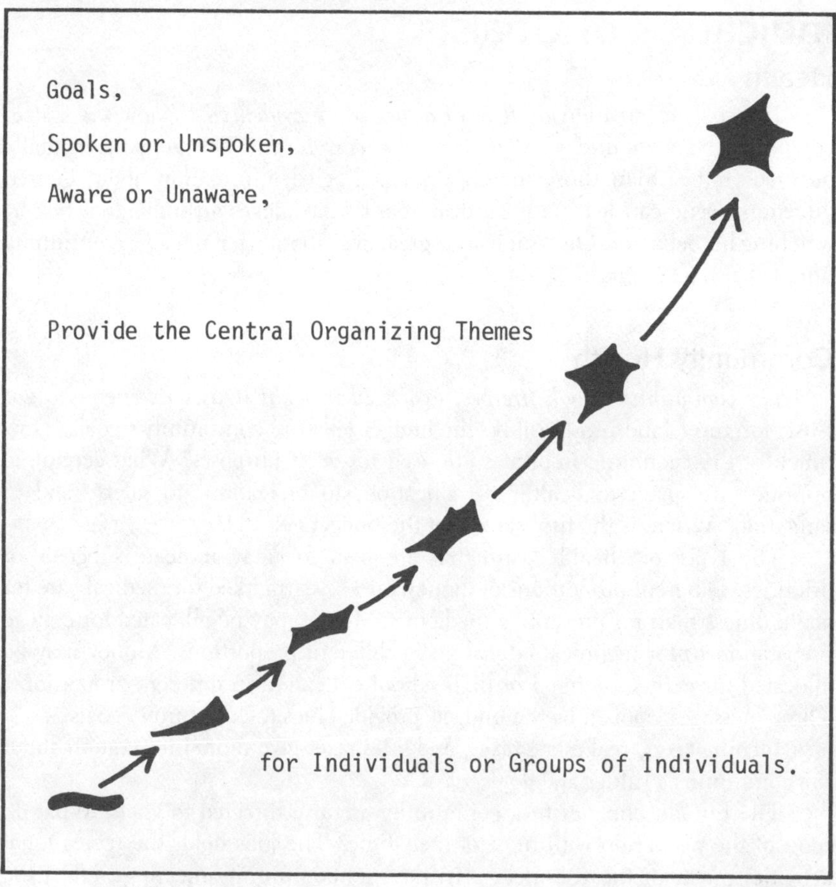
Goals,
Spoken or Unspoken,
Aware or Unaware,
Provide the Central Organizing Themes
for Individuals or Groups of Individuals.

to all members of the community, hold the people together. Minor goals and counter-goals exist in counterpoint to each other, and may be drawn together by the major themes should a need arise.

Community Health Assessment

What are the community goals that contribute to the unique character of the community? Why do people live there? What brought them to this place: a job; security; a good education for children; closeness to nature—or protection from buffeting of nature, closeness to other family members, or some other quality of the place? What keeps them here? What do they like, and what don't they like about living here? Answers to these questions will provide clues to the themes and counter-themes of the community's goals.

Indicators of Goals

Health

The goals of an individual or of a group are evidenced by how the system organizes its energy and what it uses its energy to do. The activities actually pursued, rather than those merely discussed, give information about desired directions. One can learn a great deal about what makes an individual tick by watching his behavior. One can learn a great deal about what makes a community unique by watching its behavior (Jacobs, 1961).

Community Health

The community's goals are best expressed in what it uses its energy to do. First, foremost, and most visibly, the budget tells the community's goals. How much of the economic resources are used for what purposes? What economic priorities are given to health, to education, to recreation, to safety, and to sanitation? Where is the first place that the budget gets cut?

The types of "health" care that are paid for may indicate subgoals or priorities. Different proportions of money may be earmarked for medical care for acute illness than for preventive medicine. Money may be allocated for college preparation or for technical education in different proportions. Money may be allocated for early childhood or high school education in different proportions. These messages, spoken by the budget, provide clues to community goals.

Income taxes, real estate taxes, and sales taxes give more information about the community's values and goals.

The human energies in a community are also directed to goals. What do most of the people do with most of their time? The jobs held, the recreational activities pursued, the volunteer activities and community meetings reflect the goals and subgoals of the community and its members.

The level of community health can be seen from the ways a community spends its human, economic, and political energies. Communities whose major energies are spent in safety and survival efforts enjoy a lesser level of development than communities whose energies are expended in education, caring, and other altruistic activities. In reality, energies are divided into different proportions and distributed to different tasks and different areas. It is the proportional allocation of resources to survival and safety needs, developmental needs, and altruistic activities that indicates the level of community development and provides clues to the uniqueness of the community as a whole.

Community Health Assessment

What does the community use its energies to achieve? What relative proportions of the budget go to safety and survival needs? What relative proportions of the budget go toward helping people to grow? Which parts of the city receive the major portion of the allocations? Which parts receive the least—the areas with

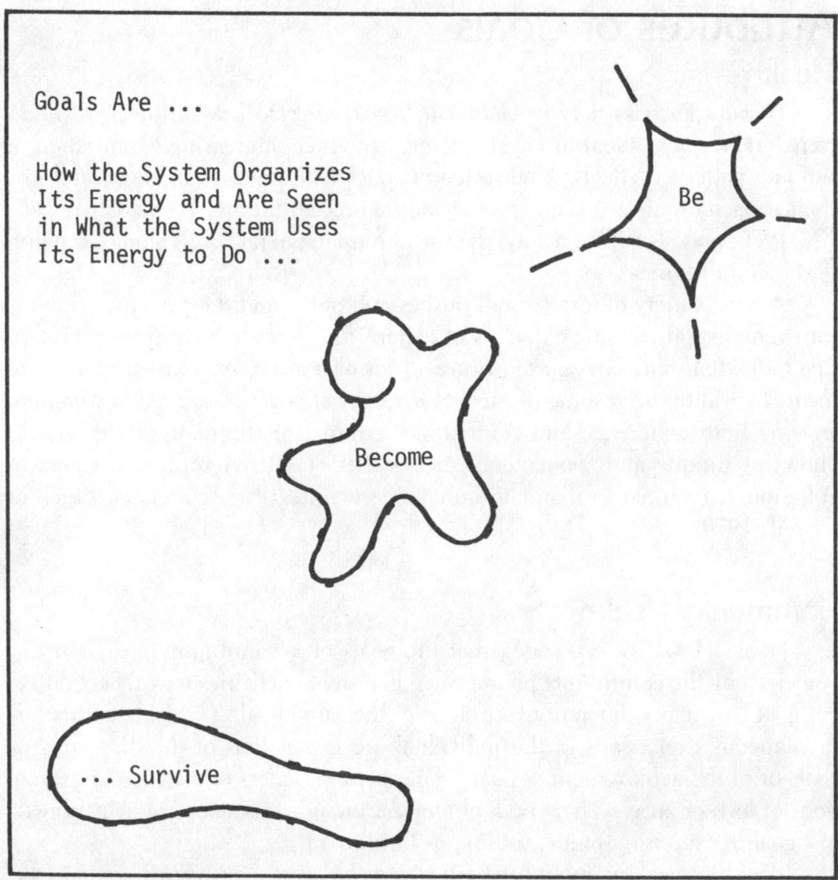
Goals Are ...
How the System Organizes Its Energy and Are Seen in What the System Uses Its Energy to Do ...
Be
Become
... Survive

greater need, or those with less need? How much does this tell you about the community's unspoken goals?

What do the people do with their free time? Watch television, attend meetings, share with others in some way? Do they take on a second job, help their children with homework, go out and have fun? What is the meaning, spoken and unspoken, of such activities?

Attributes of Goals

Health

Human energies may be channelled, goal directed (negentropic), or undirected (entropic). Goal-directed energies produce increasingly nonrandom, unique, patterned effects. Undirected energies tend toward sameness, and lose their capacity to do work, unless they are redirected toward some goal (Rogers, M., 1970, pp. 54–52). In reality, the use of human energies falls along the points of this continuum.

A wide variety of forces (both pushes and pulls) and their relative valences (or strengths) provide the elements of pattern for the individual (Lewin, 1964). *The individual may be open to (aware of) his own goals, or closed (unaware) of them.* In reality, he is some of each. A *diversity of goals is required to stimulate growth.* Both coherence and conflict are required to stimulate growth and to allow for unique and spontaneous expressions of self. A sufficient degree of cohesion is required to maintain coherence or integrity (Aguilera, Messick & Farrell, 1970).

Community Health

Jacobs (1961, p. 25) stated that the goals of a community are often not perceived by the community planners. A diversity of activities may reflect different goals, or many different expressions of the same goal. The truly authentic, spontaneous expressions of the individual are expressions of the directions of goals or of the achievement of goals. They seek closeness or distance in expressions of love or anger. They speak of progress toward, frustration, or achievement of a goal in expression of joy, futility, or fulfillment.

Goal-directed community activities may be overt or covert. They may be formally expressed in city plans, struggled through at community meetings in open expressions of their content. Less apparent goals are seen in other ways. The activities on the street, in the corner grocery store, or in the bars tell of the "covert"—but no less real—community goals.

Point and counterpoint of goals within the subsystems of a large urban area offer diversity and some of the uniqueness of a city's pattern. New York City's Times Square area offers theater and draws in the affluent who seek the entertainment, the stimulation, and perhaps the status of seeing the latest play. It offers a wide variety of ethnic restaurants, and in spite of concerted efforts by the city to "clean it up," it offers a community to professionals in pornography.

Both coherence and conflict are required to maintain integrity and to stimulate growth in communities. Goals (both pushes and pulls—or more formally, goals of avoidance and goals of desire) produce a community pattern of point and counterpoint. A community, totally united by a negative goal (such as the Klu Klux Klan), will never grow more humanistic unless some conflict, or diversity of goals, is introduced into the system. There are many less dramatic forms of

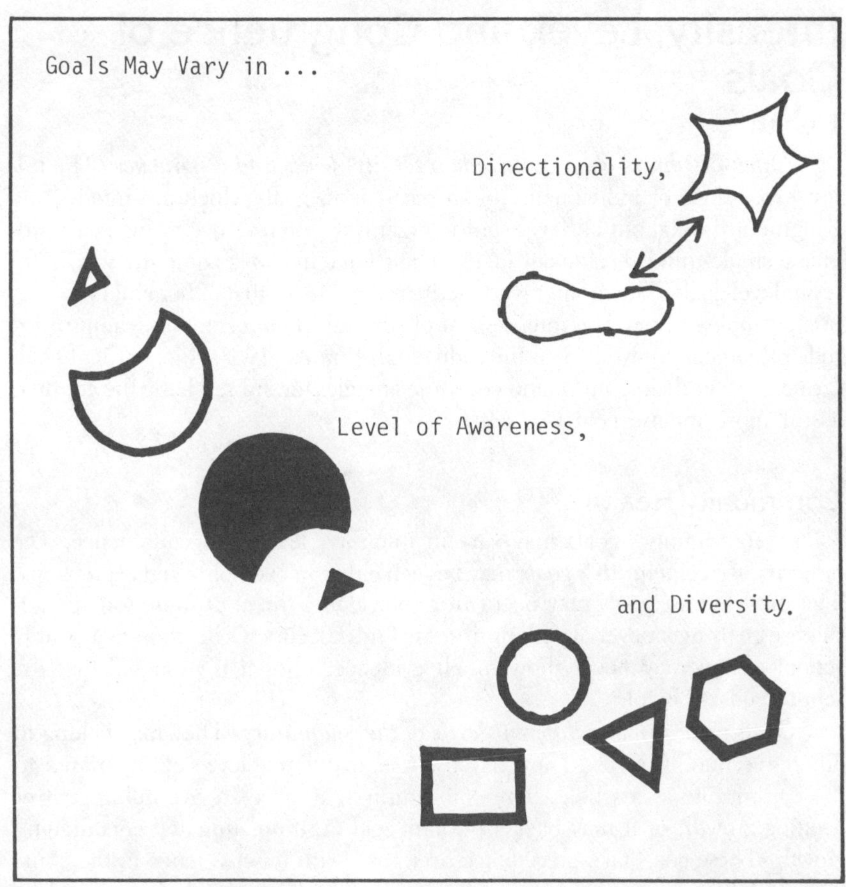
Goals May Vary in ...
Directionality,
Level of Awareness,
and Diversity.

overriding negative goals in communities—fear of a different racial or ethnic group; fear of violence; fear of families with children who swear; fear of children skilled in emotionally rich "Black English" rather than intellectually precise "White English," for example.

Community Health Assessment

What are the overt goals of the community? What are the covert goals within the community? How many different goals of point and counterpoint can you identify?

What are the ordered effects you see in the community? What themes recurr? What are the evidences of randomness? Are there many run-down decaying stores, neighborhoods, or groups of people? What are the causes for this?

What are the evidences of uniqueness, spontaneity, joy and whimsy in the community? How frequently do they occur?

Intensity, Level, and Congruence of Goals

Health

Other attributes of goals include intensity, level, and congruence. The fullest expressions of individuality often result from goals which are intense and congruent throughout all levels of the organism. Intense, overriding goals provide a single-minded, efficient focus. Their force may overcome the valence of lesser level goals. The mother who sacrifices her life for that of her child provides one example of this. The intense goal of survival in concentration camps overrode other goals and values of the individuals (Frankl, 1963). Incongruent goals create stress in the organism and consume energies toward resolving the conflict, a still more intense goal in itself.

Community Health

A community's goals may vary in intensity, level, and congruence. *The intensity of a community's goals* may be seen either in overt or covert expressions. The most intense goals may occur in response to a threat of some sort. Quiet, intense goals may never appear until some "rub" occurs. Dedication to a quality school system may never show much evidence, until it is proposed that the school budget be cut.

Goals exist at many different levels of the community. They may belong to different economic levels. They may also refer to different levels of importance to the community as a whole. The community may have an overriding goal of limiting growth, or it may have a primary goal of stimulating and encouraging growth. These goals take precedence over goals with lesser valence in the community. Setting priorities is one method used to make the level of goals explicit and visible.

Goals in a community may vary in regard to their congruence (goodness of fit) with each other (Alexander, 1964). Acute community stresses may result from intense, incongruent goals. Chronic, low-grade community stress may result from less intense, incongruent goals. Differing goals across differing levels of the community may create either acute or chronic community stresses.

One indicator of a community's level of wellness is its ability to differentiate, articulate, and resolve or accept the conflicting goals of its members.

Alinsky (1969) proposed a strategy for resolution of conflicting goals by identifying an overriding, more intense, higher level goal which *is* congruent between the groups. This goal is then used as a common bond and provides a stronger valence for the resolution of the conflict.

The most visible (or audible) conflicting goals in a community are related to the allocation of scarce resources. Dollars, space, personnel, and services are often sought for special programs by special interest groups. Legislative or municipal hearings provide a means for presenting the issues and the needs involved. Through the mechanism of open democratic government, optimum resolution

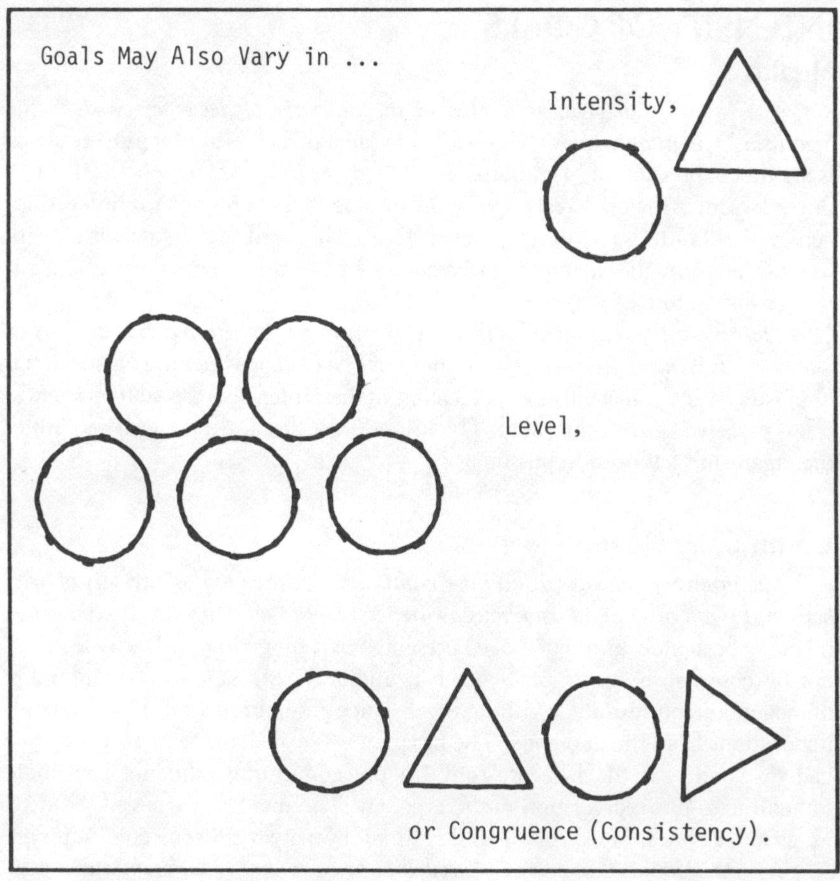
Goals May Also Vary in ...
Intensity,
Level,
or Congruence (Consistency).

and resource allocation can occur. It is certainly evident that through hearing all sides of an issue, new ideas, and aspects of a problem can be differentiated.

Community Health Assessment

What types of goals are most intensely felt in the community at present? What local issues make headlines, appear as letters to the editor, or occur during conversations between friends?

What are the levels of goals involved? Are they goals that affect the community as a whole, or that affect smaller groups within the community? Are they goals that are primary, and override lesser goals?

What are the incongruent goals within the community? Does the community want to increase its growth but not spend any money for increasing the capacity of the school system?

INTENSITY OF GOALS

Health

The intensity of goals is related to the intensity of need perceived by the organism. The intensity with which an individual perceives and/or pursues a goal is another expression of his uniqueness. The perceived need may be related to a direct lack of a material resource, of an unweighted energy, or to the need for achievement of the next developmental level. The need may be perceived with full awareness by the organism, or be perceived as only a vague sense of uneasiness or discomfort.

The amount of free energy which the organism has to perceive its goals may or may not affect their intensity. The amount of free energy which the organism has to pursue its goals may affect its perception of their intensity. A goal looses power if it is perceived as unachievable. The loss of hope, for a specific goal will buffer the organism's felt need to pursue it.

Community Health

The intensity of goals within the community is related to the intensity of need perceived (with or without conscious awareness) by the community. The community may be acutely aware of a need presented by a program cut. It may feel, but not be consciously aware of, a need in another area. In one very culturally homogenous community, a visiting Black dance group brought numerous standing ovations from the audience. The program was excellent, to be sure, but one had to wonder, if the lack of "soul" in the community, did not contribute something to the appreciation of the program. The incident suggested the need for greater richness of expression and cultural diversity within the community.

A *certain amount of energy is needed to perceive and to differentiate a goal.* Individuals must be able to attend to the need, groups must be able to meet to discuss—and thereby differentiate and clarify—the goal. This requires available energies of time; interest; transportation; meeting space; personal energies of the organizers and the attenders; media time/space; and baby sitters; etc. A goal must have sufficient valence (perceived need plus perceived achievability) in the first place to draw that much energy from the community. One of the functions of community is the presence of preexisting resources and networks, so that less energy will be required for such efforts.

Community meeting spaces, informal baby-sitting services, a consistent space in the newspaper to announce community meetings are all methods which both signify a certain level of development in the community and enhance its ability to perceive and pursue the goals of its people and groups.

The amount of free energy which the organism has to pursue the goal may increase the valence (power) of that goal, especially if it is a conscious goal. Unconscious, or only half-conscious goals may be pursued just as vigorously, if the community has sufficient available energy to do so. "Burnt out" communities, hopeless communities, may have little available energy to pursue

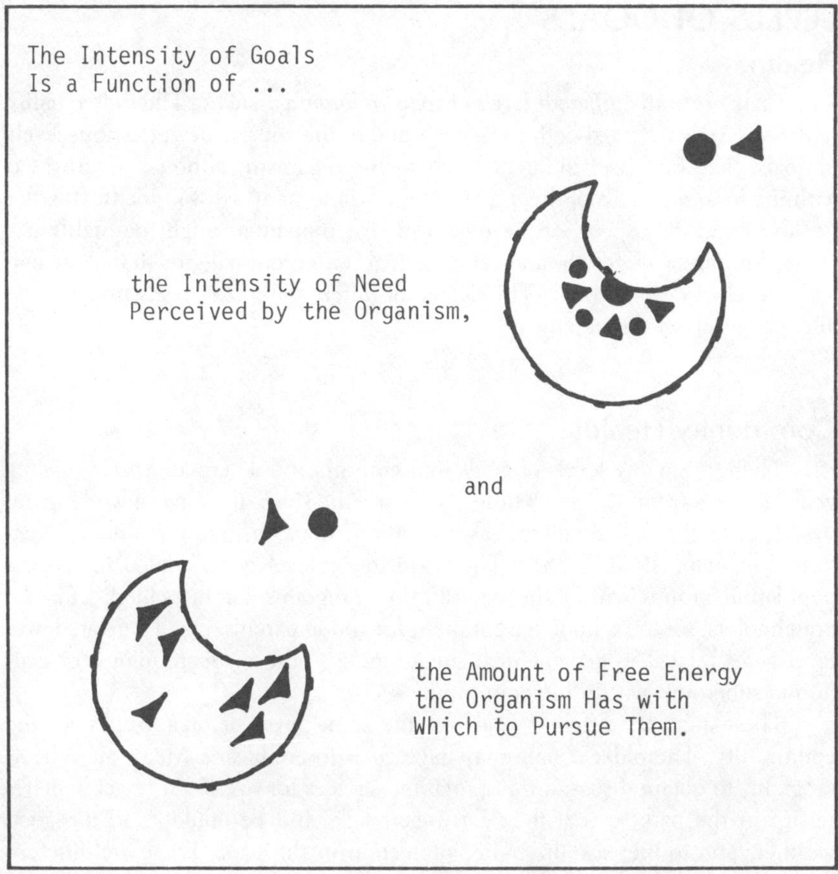
The Intensity of Goals
Is a Function of ...
the Intensity of Need
Perceived by the Organism,
and
the Amount of Free Energy
the Organism Has with
Which to Pursue Them.

goals, and lose the power to achieve them. Communities bound to conflicting goals may have little free energy left to pursue goals outside of "winning" or resolving intracommunity or community-suprasystem conflict. They thereby lose some of their capacity to expend the energy required for unique and spontaneous expressions of self.

Community Health Assessment

What are the current most acutely felt needs and goals within the community? What energies will be required for the community to pursue them? Which of these energies are available in the community? Which are not presently available? What can the community do to increase its access to the necessary energies? What energies can be released from other tasks to the pursuit of these goals?

LEVELS OF GOALS

Health

There are many different levels of goals in human systems. The individuality of the system is reflected both in its goals and in the consistency of various levels of goals. The health of different levels of the organism, although intertwined with the level of health of the organism as a whole, may assist in identifying the health of specific aspects of the organism. An individual might be highly developed in physical growth, and yet have goals for emotional growth that are at a lesser level of development. The degree of differentiation of goals may vary at different levels of the organism.

Community Health

There are many levels of goals in a community. There are the overriding goals of the community as a whole. There are the subgoals, ways of working out overall goals through smaller areas: education, housing, transportation, recreation (Freeman, 1970, p. 61). There are lower level goals related to specific population groups within the community. Programs for the elderly, for the preschoolers, for the school-age children, for young parents, etc. There are lower level goals related to geographical subgroupings, ethnic subgroupings, or economic subgroups within the community.

There may be different goals on the same level of organization of the community. The older people may have goals to establish a Meals on Wheels program, to obtain discount transportation services for over 65's, to get benches set up in the park so that they can meet, talk, and be outdoors in the good weather, and to increase the police protection in the park. These are different goals of one level (identified by age group) of the community.

Goals of different economic levels of the community might include goals around the issue of bussing children to school. These goals might be congruent—if both the economically advantaged and the economically disadvantaged approve of bussing. If both groups want to stop the bussing, this is still a congruent goal.

Both the economically advantaged group and the economically disadvantaged groups might want to see a new industry come into town in order to obtain jobs and tax relief.

The level of health of a community is reflected in its goals. Goals related to simple survival needs may be the overt, overriding goals of the community as a whole (especially in economically depressed communities). Survival level goals may be held by some groups within the community, while other goals are held by the community as a whole. Altruistic goals may be those of the community as a whole, or only one or more subgroups within the community. Service agencies and clubs often have more or less well-differentiated altruistic goals.

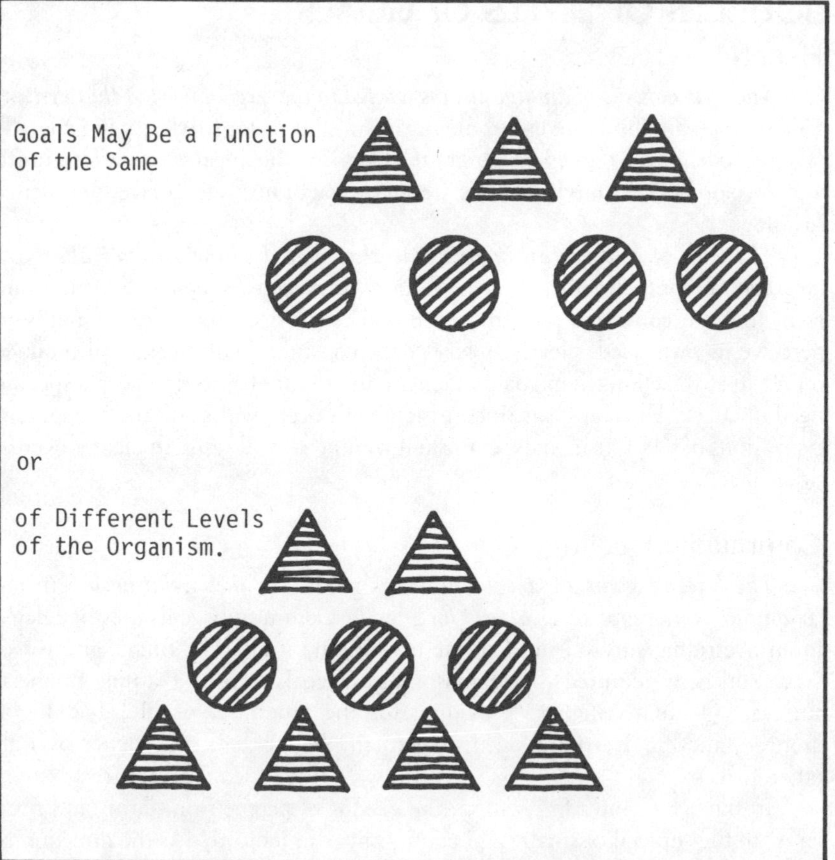

Goals May Be a Function
of the Same
or
of Different Levels
of the Organism.

Community Health Assessment

One of the steps in community health assessment is identifying the level to which a given goal belongs. Conversely, identifying the goals of different levels of the community aids in assessing the level of wellness of the whole, and of the specific sub-systems within the community.

What are the goals of the different age groups in the community? What are the goals of the different economic groups within the community? What are the goals of the major providers of different services within the community?

SOURCES OF LEVELS OF GOALS

Health

The level of goals of an organism is related to the level of need of that system. Goals which are fundamental to the organism's needs for survival will generally take precedence over goals which are related to the organism's needs for growth and development. If survival needs are met, growth needs then take precedence (Maslow, 1955).

The level of goals in an organism is also related to the system's ability to incorporate inputs, whether of weighted or of unweighted energies. Stated, aware goals that are consistent with the need will result from the system's ability to perceive its own needs clearly. Clear goals, consistent with need, will produce more effective actions than goals which are the result of a need to keep a specific need in check. Unclear goals, inconsistent with need, will result in incongruent expressions of self. Clear goals, consistent with need, will result in clearer expressions of self.

Community Health

The level of goals in a community is related to their relationship to the community's needs for survival and for growth. Community goals may be related to an overriding survival need of the community itself. The financial crisis of New York City required the establishment of goals to assure simple financial survival. Qualitative goals, providing for the amenities of life, had to be dropped, and the overriding need to maintain the city took precedence over all other goals.

In the age of industrialization, the exodus of people from farms and rural land put the survival of small rural communities in jeopardy. As the direction of flow of human energy reverses, and families move out from the city to suburban and rural areas, the survival and quality of cities is endangered. Assuring the survival of a community, maintaining the minimum functions for the health and safety of its residents, takes priority over goals related to increasing the quality of life.

Barriers to both weighted and unweighted energies affect the community's abilities to meet its needs. As a result, goals remain congruent with lesser levels of development. Urban areas have only few ways to tax the higher income members of the surrounding surburban areas which live off the jobs, the culture, the transportation, the media, and other resources provided by the city. The formal boundaries, established in an earlier age, prevent an equitable sharing of costs for maintaining the city's resources. Similarly, as the younger, more affluent families, with greater interest and concern about the quality of the school system, the accessibility of recreation space, and with the mobility and resources provided by well-paying jobs, cars, babysitters, etc., move out to the suburbs, the human energy available to solve the inner city's problems is decreased.

Boundaries, which affect the community's abilities to incorporate inputs, include the culture and values of the community. Communities with a high

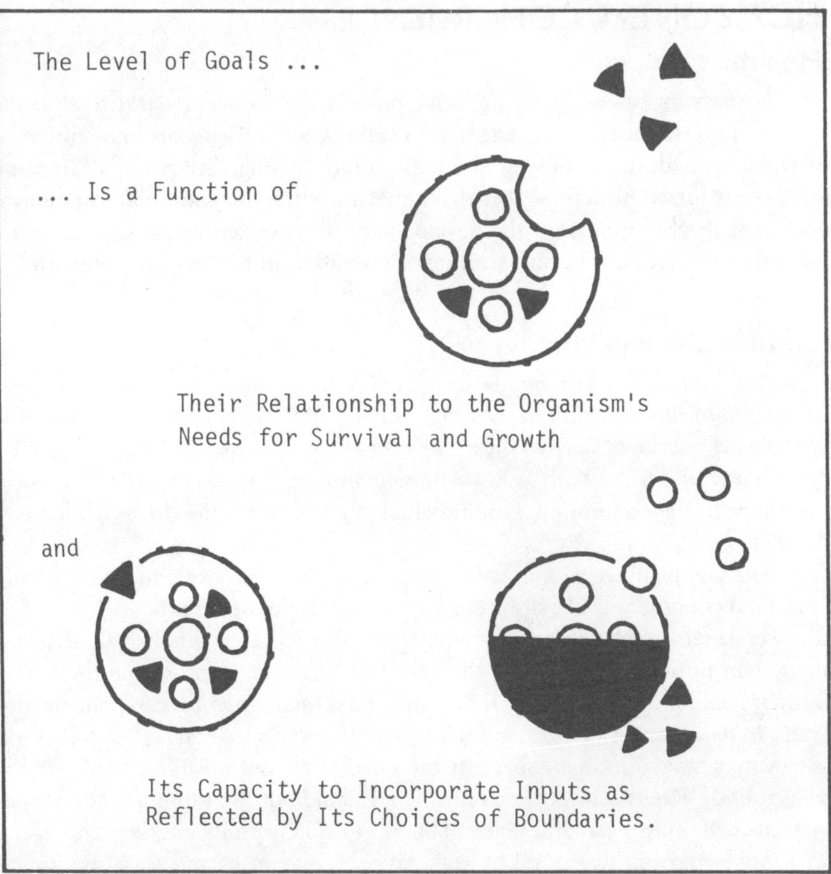

degree of closure in some area will be less able to incorporate inputs in that area, and therefore will have stronger, unmet, unconscious needs. The community which sets such a high value on "morality" that it cannot allow a sex education program in the school will have many unmet needs in developing information, attitudes, and judgments concerning teenage sexuality. A community goal to "preserve the morality of teenagers" may gain in intensity to counteract the power of the original need. Religious education programs and sports programs may gain priority as the level of unmet need increases.

The Level of Goals ...
... Is a Function of
Their Relationship to the Organism's
Needs for Survival and Growth
and
Its Capacity to Incorporate Inputs as
Reflected by Its Choices of Boundaries.

Community Health Assessment

What level of needs does the community's stated goals reflect? Are the major community goals directed toward survival, toward growth, or toward facilitation of the fullest contribution of its members?

Are the community's goals directly related to the needs of its members or are they reflections of needs which the community is unable to perceive in a direct way?

HORIZONTAL CONGRUENCE

Health

Goals may be congruent or incongruent across one horizontal level of the system. Diverse goals are necessary for health. Conflicting goals may inhibit or stimulate growth, depending on their resolution. Incongruent goals, at the same level of organization, represent such conflict and either may stimulate an innovative, new level of growth or the development of increased barriers between the two groups or areas, with the resulting deterioration in health of the organism.

Community Health

A *community's goals may be congruent or incongruent throughout one level of the organism.* A community's horizontal pattern consists of the networks, nodes, and boundaries across the same level of the community. Warren uses the term horizontal pattern "to indicate those community units insofar as they have relevance to the community system, which tend to be on the same hierarchical level" (1963, p. 162).

The city planning commission, board of aldermen, or other planning body may hold congruent goals, or be engaged in a struggle over conflicting goals. On a lower level of the city's hierarchy, small districts may hold goals that are congruent throughout the city—all areas have set increased safety on the streets as their goal for the next year. Or they may hold incongruent goals—one district wants to reduce taxes by cutting services, another wants to increase services. One group may want the open space at the edge of its district to be made into a playground. The downtown area on the other side of the same boundary may want it made into a parking space. These, obviously are incongruent goals.

Goals may be diverse, yet fit well. An open play space and a parking garage may not be incongruent if both groups can agree to the notion of an underground parking lot with play space on top. Additional caution about exhaust fumes may have to be taken. Perhaps the two groups would be willing to share the cost of providing for safety measures to control this.

The power company's perceived need, and, therefore, its goal, to maintain the use of local highways to transport radioactive materials is incongruent with the community's desire to stop the transport of these materials through the city streets. Both goals are expressions of the unique perceptions and character of the groups they represent.

The goal of stopping the transport of nuclear waste may be held by all the small communities in the state, and is, therefore, congruent at that level of the state's organization (Braun, 1977).

A community's phase of health can be seen from the congruence of its goals. Goals may be congruent, resting, awaiting new impetus, and energies may be directed toward maintaining these states. On the other hand, goals may be incongruent, and the community's efforts may be directed toward resolving the

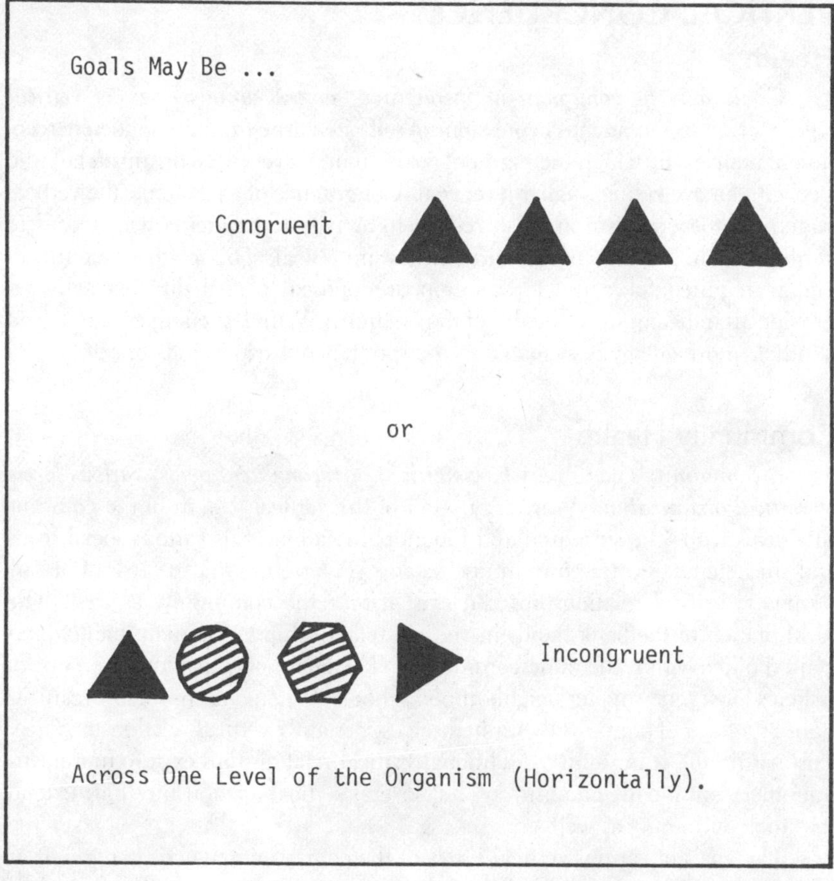
Goals May Be ...
Congruent
or
Incongruent
Across One Level of the Organism (Horizontally).

conflict between goals. Generally, of course, different phases of activity-rest are taking place at all times with regard to different areas and types of goals within a large, complex community.

Community Health Assessment

What level of the community has the most visible goals? Are they congruent or incongruent? What areas of the community are directing their energies toward the resolution of conflicting goals?

VERTICAL CONGRUENCE

Health

Goals may be congruent or incongruent across various levels of vertical organization. Spontaneous expressions of self often arise from the sudden perception of a means by which incongruent goals on one level of the organism fall into step with an overriding, higher level goal. Congruence of goals across the vertical pattern of the organism are also related to activity-rest patterns with regard to conflict resolution or activities directed toward a goal. The relative amounts of energy required for conflict resolution as opposed to goal directed activities provide an indicator of the health of the organism. With less energies bound into conflict, more energy is available to the spontaneous expressions of self.

Community Health

A *community's goals may be congruent or incongruent across various levels of vertical organization.* Warren's notion of the vertical pattern of the community deals with "the structural and functional relation of its various social units and subsystems to extra-community systems" (Warren, 1963, p. 161). For our purposes, vertical relationships can exist *within* the community as well. The local branch of the bank stands in vertical relationship to the main branch and central office within the same community. The board of education may control policies for several smaller neighborhood schools. When one considers organizations as a form of community in themselves, certainly vertical relationships may exist within the community. Additional vertical relationships exist to more central offices outside the community, but several vertical relationships may extend into the community as well.

The goals of various vertical levels of the community may be congruent or incongruent. The local school district may be in conflict with the board of education regarding the qualifications of teachers, the content of, or approaches to, education. The sensitivity of teachers to the needs of the children as opposed to their educational qualifications may be at issue. The "return to basics" as opposed to stimulation of intellectual curiosity and competence in affective or interpersonal skills may be at issue. These are issues about which both parents and educators hold strong opinions (Brown, 1971; Hentoff, 1966; Illich, 1970).

Conflicting vertical goals may be resolved in several ways: from the top down (Milgram, 1974), *from the bottom up, or from some compromise between the two.* A unilateral decision or resolution, will, of course, leave the pressures from the unmet needs of the "other" side of the issue unresolved. Literal or figurative sabbotage will, of necessity, result, unless it is the "straw that breaks the camel's back" and results in apathy—a no-win "success."

Where strong conflicts exist, organization of the basic power of the lower levels within a vertical hierarchy—the energies of the numbers of people involved—can be used to balance the force of power. This is the principle underlying unionization, work stoppages, slowdowns, strikes, demonstrations, and political letter writing campaigns.

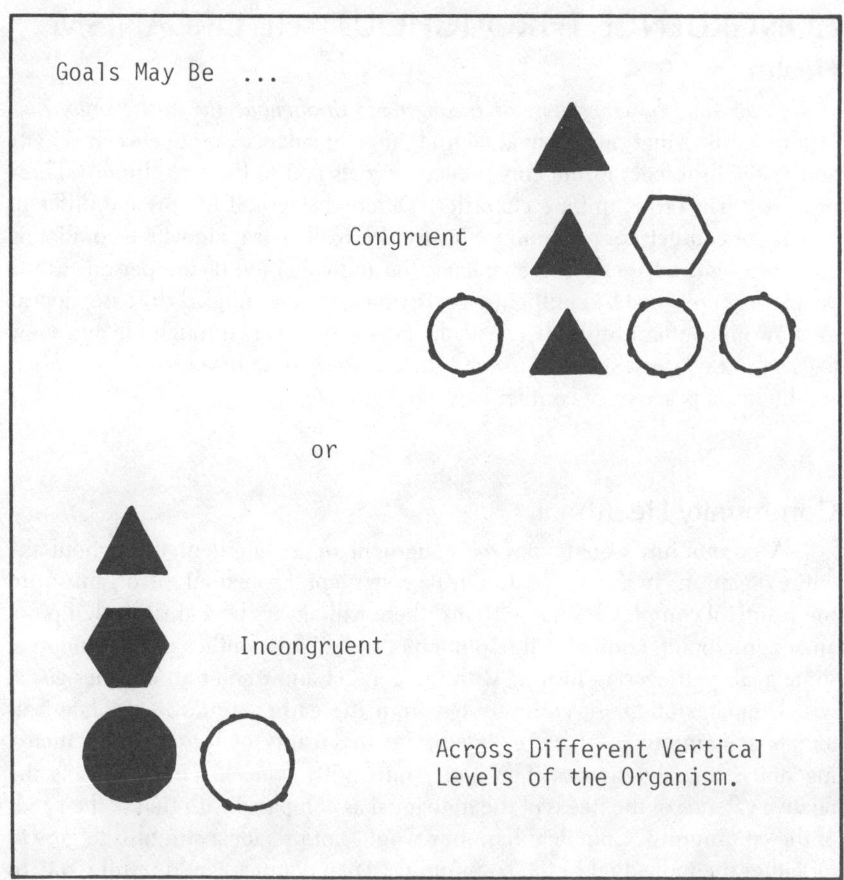
Goals May Be ...
Congruent
or
Incongruent
Across Different Vertical
Levels of the Organism.

Community Health Assessment

What are the conflicting goals across different vertical levels of the community? What have been the *successful* strategies for conflict resolution in the past? What have been the *unsuccessful* strategies for conflict resolution in the past? What is the community's traditional approach to vertical conflict of goals? Has this been a success, or not? In what ways?

CONGRUENCE THROUGHOUT THE ORGANISM

Health

Goals may be congruent or incongruent throughout the entire organism. Health requires that each individual find the right balance point between activity and rest with respect to the congruence of goals and to their resolution. These provide a part of his unique character. Different stages of life present different "crises" or conflicts for resolution (Sheehy, 1976). The ways in which conflicting goals are resolved marks the character (the individuality) of the person. Some people seem plagued by conflicting goals; others, single-minded, intense, appear to know no conflict. Still others placidly pursue their way through life and show few signs of conflict. Most of us have known some time in our own lives when conditions of peace or of conflict have predominated.

Community Health

A community's goals may be congruent or incongruent throughout the entire organism. In theory, goals may be congruent throughout the organism. In the reality of complex human systems, there will always be a great deal of point and counterpoint, conflict and resolution of goals. This conflict and resolution of some goals will overlap in time with the conflict and resolution of other goals.

Utopian notions of community—from the earliest times to the latest attempts at communes—have collided with the reality of human spontaneity, ingenuity, and differences. The basic, nitty-gritty issue in community is the relative valence of the needs of the individual as compared with that of the needs of the community. Complete harmony would not provide a stimulus to growth for either the individual or the community. Total conflict would result in chaos and the overriding of either the needs of the individual or the needs of the group. No energies would be available to the pursuit of other tasks.

The relative amount of harmony and conflict of goals within a community is a response to the unique internal and external pressures the community undergoes. One would think, that, in general, communities with abundant resources, accessible to all, would undergo less conflict than communities with scarcer resources. However, an exception to this is seen in nontechnologically oriented communities, in which all resources, whether abundant or scarce, are shared by all members of the community.

One aspect of a community's individuality is its methods for dealing with conflict. Vermont town meetings encourage and allow the expressions of diverse interests. Legislative hearings and reaction papers also encourage this. Totalitarian countries discourage the expression of diverse interests and approaches. Some communities allow, and neither encourage nor discourage, the expression of diverse interests. They are simply accepted, and permitted to occur.

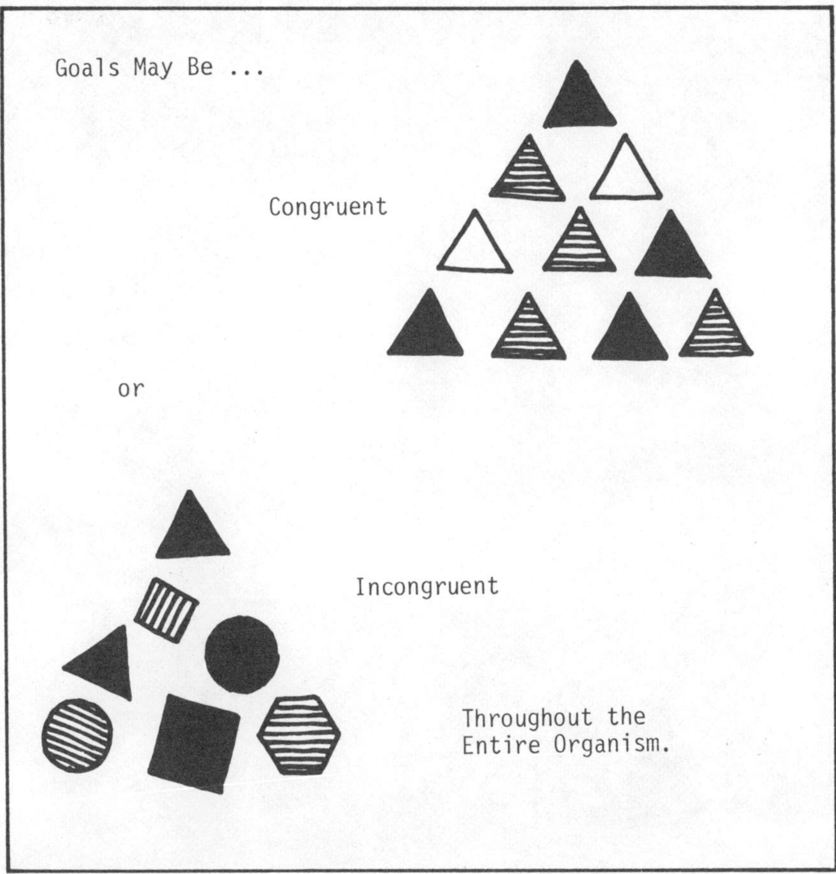
Goals May Be ...
Congruent
or
Incongruent
Throughout the
Entire Organism.

Community Health Assessment

What is the relative balance of congruent and incongruent goals within the community? What is the need for conflict resolution? Is the community being torn by conflict, or is it apathetic and passively denying the existence of conflict? Does it encourage conflict or discourage it? What are the current issues involved?

References and Resources

REFERENCES

Aguilera, Donna, Messick, Janice, & Farrell, Marlene. *Crisis Intervention: Theory and Methodology*. St. Louis: C. V. Mosby, 1970.

Alexander, Christopher. *Notes on the Synthesis of Form*. Cambridge, Mass.: Harvard University, 1964.

Alinsky, Saul. *Reveille for Radicals*. New York: Vintage, 1969.

Braun, Bill. Vermonters resist nuclear power. *The Burlington Free Press*, March 2, 1977, p. 1.

Brown, George. *Human Teaching for Human Learning: An Introduction to Confluent Education*. New York: Viking, 1971.

Frankl, Viktor. *Man's Search for Meaning: An Introduction to Logotherapy*. New York: Washington Square, 1963.

Freeman, Ruth. *Community Health Nursing Practice*. Philadelphia: W. B. Saunders, 1970.

Hentoff, Nat. *Our Children are Dying*. New York: Viking, 1966.

Illich, Ivan. *Deschooling Society*. New York: Harper & Row, 1970.

Jacobs, Jane. *The Death and Life of Great American Cities*. New York: Vintage, 1961.

Lewin, Kurt. *Field Theory in Social Science: Selected Theoretical Papers*. New York: Harper, 1964.

Maslow, Abraham. Deficiency motivation and growth motivation. In Marshall Jones (Ed.), *Nebraska Symposium on Motivation*, 3, 1–30. Lincoln: University of Nebraska Press, 1955.

Maslow, Abraham. *Toward a Psychology of Being*. Princeton: D. Van Nostrand, 1962.

Milgram, Stanley. *Obedience to Authority: An Experimental View:* New York: Harper & Row, 1974.

Rogers, Martha. *An Introduction to the Theoretical Basis of Nursing*. Philadelphia: F. A. Davis, 1970.

Schloltfeldt, Rozella. Personal communication, 1974.

Sheehy, Gail. *Passages: Predictable Crises of Adult Life*. New York: Bantam, 1976.

Warren, Roland. *The Community in America*. Chicago: Rand McNally, 1963.

RESOURCES

Buhler, Charlotte. The life cycle: structural determinants of goal setting. *The Journal of Humanistic Psychology*, 1966, 6, 37–52.

Teilhard de Chardin, Pierre. *The Phenomenon of Man*. New York: Harper, 1959.

Illich, Ivan. *Medical Nemesis*. London: Marion Boyars, 1975.

Kallen, Horace. Innovation. In Amatia Etzioni & Eva Etzioni-Halevy (Eds.), *Social Change: Sources, Patterns and Consequences*. (Second edition.) New York: Basic Books, 1973. pp. 447–450.

Maslow, Abraham. *The Farther Reaches of Human Nature*. New York: Viking, 1971.

May, Rollo. *Love and Will*. New York: W. W. Norton, 1969.

Pelletier, Kenneth. *Mind as Healer, Mind as Slayer*. New York: Delta, 1977.

Satir, Virginia. *Peoplemaking*. Palo Alto, Calif.: Science and Behavior, 1972.

Sparer, Gerald, Dines, George, & Smith, Daniel. Consumer participation in OEO-assisted neighborhood health centers. *American Journal of Public Health*, 1970, *60*, 1091–1102.

6

CHAPTER SIX

Organization: The Forces and Functions of Goals

Organization of a community results from the forces activated by its goals. The goals may have been past goals, now frozen in formal or organizational structures. The goals may be future goals, creating pressures for change of such structures.

Goals provide the push and pull which create, maintain, or change pattern. Perception of organization requires perception of forces driving in the same or different directions. Organization gives dimensions of time and motion to the community's pattern. The description of the community's organization requires recognition of the forces which direct the energies of the community and its people.

Initiating Forces

Health

The congruence of goals is a function of the organism's ability to perceive and pursue its goals. Any system must be able to perceive its own needs accurately in order to be able to pursue them. Boundaries function as walls to perception (Eriksen, 1951) and thereby blind the organism to its own needs and goals. Boundaries, by blinding the organism to its own needs, blind it to the goals it has wittingly or unwittingly established to meet these needs. Conflicting goals, therefore, are not perceived as such.

Conflicting goals may also produce or reinforce already existing boundaries. Conflicting goals may be seen, by both sides of the division, as cause, or further cause, for barricading against the "other." Any human system must be able eventually to see across its boundaries, if it is to grow.

Community Health

The congruence of a community's goals is a function of its ability to perceive and pursue its own needs. In a community with tight boundaries, the people on one side of the tracks cannot perceive the needs of the people on the other side of the tracks. The impact of the severe needs reaches across the borders, but their causes cannot be accurately perceived, and therefore no appropriate actions can be designed. The impact of the problem becomes attributed to a vague, undifferentiated blame, attributed to the "other people." The specific reason for this "otherness" of the groups is irrelevant. However, it becomes the focus of perceived relevance. It becomes the foundation for the boundary's walls, and, as such, has great value to those who need the boundary to remain secure. Ethnicity, economics, lack of emphasis on traditional approaches can all serve as nebulous support for a rigid boundary.

It is best not to challenge the boundary itself; rather, strategies to bypass, hurdle, hop over, or go around the boundary in the smallest, least threatening ways serve better (network building). The support provided by the boundary is necessary, until it no longer fills a need.

A community must be able to see across its boundaries if it is to grow. Barriers to accurate perception or empathy prevent the community from recognizing its total needs, and from planning strategies to meet these needs without raising conflict with their root causes.

Some attempts at planning have aimed at blasting through boundaries—for instance, consumer participation, at whatever level (Arnstein, 1969), has not been overwhelmingly successful. The otherness, rather than the togetherness, has often increased. Misperceptions and misunderstandings are the basic bricks from which boundaries and walls are built and maintained. They can best be removed by small, committed, precise attempts to clarify each issue (Bennis, Benne & Chin, 1969).

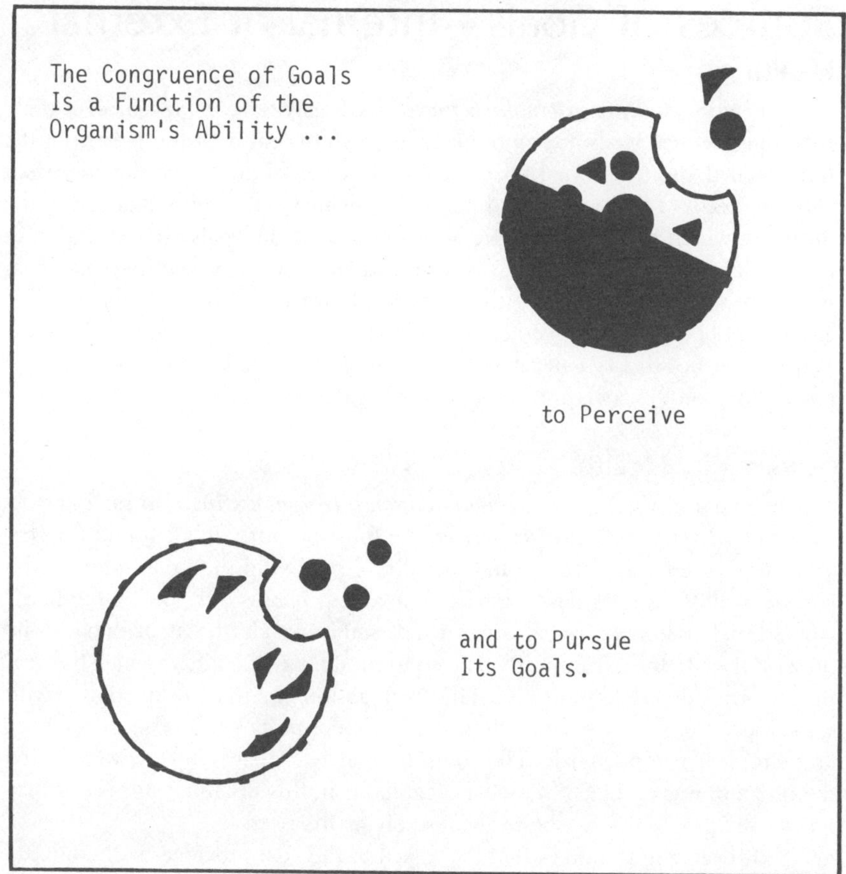
The Congruence of Goals
Is a Function of the
Organism's Ability ...
to Perceive
and to Pursue
Its Goals.

A healthy, growing community needs to have leaders who are willing to peek over the boundaries, see clearly the issues on the other side, and report back. Conversations, hearing the other openly and speaking to be heard, are all required for growth.

Community Health Assessment

What incongruent goals in the community are the result of boundaries? What needs are represented by these goals? How can they be interpreted to the other side in such a way as to be heard? How well can the community perceive its own goals? How well is it able to mobilize its members to pursue them?

Sources of Goals—Internal or External

Health

Either internally or externally perceived needs may serve as the sources of goals. Internally defined goals are more likely to be consistent with the pattern of the individual than are external goals. However, external goals may be consistent with the needs of the system, and internal goals may reflect only that part of the organism which the system is able to perceive. Healthy goals are not always in perfect harmony with the system's current pattern, but may require reorganization or repatterning to occur. At some point, however, even externally imposed goals must be internally accepted, or resistance, sabotage, or apathy will occur. Whether or not this is a negative factor in health depends upon the particular goal, and upon the goals and values of the organism.

Community Health

A *community's goals may originate from intrinsic, extrinsic, or some combination of intrinsic and extrinsic sources.* An internal source of a community goal arises from the felt need of an individual or group within the community who perceives, differentiates, and expresses a goal as a means of resolving the need. An external source of a goal arises when some outside threat or opportunity presents itself to the community. The community may then incorporate the goal into its own value system, or accept the goal, although it remains in conflict with some aspects of its own value system. Government-proposed bussing systems are an example of external goals. The community may or may not perceive the need the program was designed to meet (integration, in this instance). It may or may not see the proposal as the best way of resolving the need.

However, the resources that are linked to the goal provided by the outside source may override the unresolved conflict.

The chronic, unresolved conflict in this instance becomes a constant source of stress to the community, and, once again, may result in pressure toward a more successful resolution of the conflict, or a nagging drain on the community's energies and an additional source of stress to its people.

A healthy community is able to perceive and express its own needs and goals. It is able to evaluate the congruence and potential value of externally presented goals in relation to its own needs and goals. In general, internally identified goals are more consistent with the community's needs and pattern, and represent the next developmental need more accurately than an externally defined goal. Externally defined goals are more likely to originate from a central source and relate to several communities, and therefore no account is taken of the uniqueness of each particular community involved.

Community Health Assessment

What are the major internal sources of goals in the community? What are the major external sources of goals? Which goals are most consistent with the unique pattern of the community?

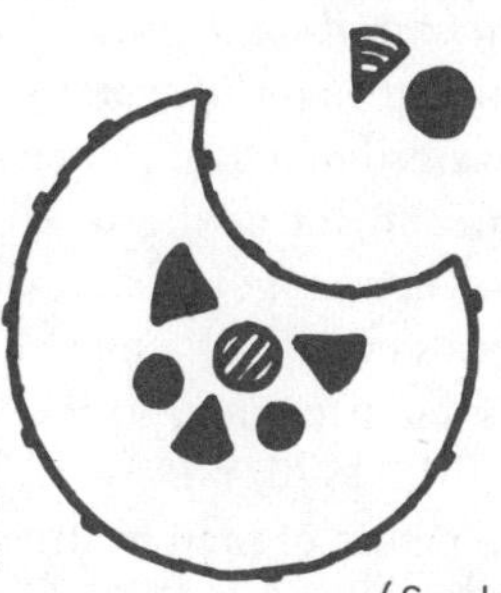
Internal Goals,
Rooted in and Resulting from the Same Unique Source Are Likely to be Congruent with Internal Patterns
(Such as DNA and RNA).

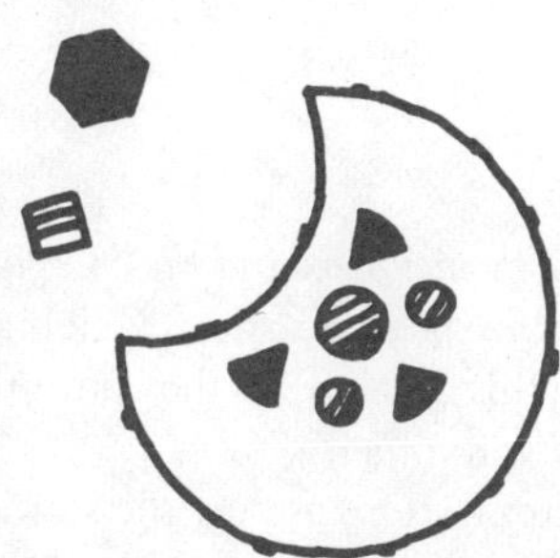
External Goals,
Originating the Other Unique, but Different Sources Are More Likely to Be Incongruent with Internal Goals and Patterns.

Synchronization of Goals

Health

Congruent goals pull energies into synchronization, and, by such coherence, exhibit a new and powerful energy (synergy). Once a human system has perceived a need and agreed to a goal to meet that need—whether as a sudden, spontaneous phenomenon, or as the result of a long and tiresome struggle to achieve consensus—a new surge of energy in pursuit of the goal is felt. Generally, new needs and goals emerge at a higher level of organization, they are perceived and resolved at some pace, and so it continues (Chermayeff & Alexander, 1965, p. 142; Rogers, M., 1970, pp. 99–101).

It is the nature of man to strive toward the next goal, as well as to savor the goals he has achieved before going on. Alpha rhythms in brain activity are associated with the physiology of satisfaction (Parmeggiani, 1968). Those who achieve alpha states in meditation perceive the rest and delight of goalessness, and feel as if they are perched on the point between goal seeking and satisfaction (Deikman, in Tart, 1969, pp. 23–43).

Community Health

Congruent community goals pull the energies of its members and the energies of the resources at the command of its members into synchronization. Celebrations and holidays provide for a means of exercising this capacity, as the community organizes to celebrate and share its celebration with others.

Acute survival threats pull energies into synchronization, as does the slower process of working through acceptance and consensus of some specific priority or plan. The process of rest and goal-seeking behaviors occur in rhythms (balanced or unbalanced rhythms) and their pace reflects the community's organization.

There is a "high" associated with the sharing, the extra energy, the heightened sense of community which is perceived by all and consciously shared by all in the pursuit of common goals.

The energy resulting from congruent goals in community can be seen at any level of need. Survival and safety needs, when attacked, pull people together into a working harmony. Floods, earthquakes, or other natural disasters may produce this phenomenon. The first East Coast blackout resulted in several hours of independent New Yorkers efficiently pulling together and getting high from the energy and empathy that resulted. During the Second World War, when it was announced that all Jews should wear arm bands in order for others to identify them, the King of Denmark went on his morning ride with an arm band on, and soon the population of the entire country was wearing arm bands with the star of David on them. This innovative, creative approach, altruistic in its source, pulled all the energies of the people into harmony, and into a very effective strategy.

Strikes, demonstrations, and other approaches yet to be devised, are evidences of the synchronization of human energies to a single purpose. Family

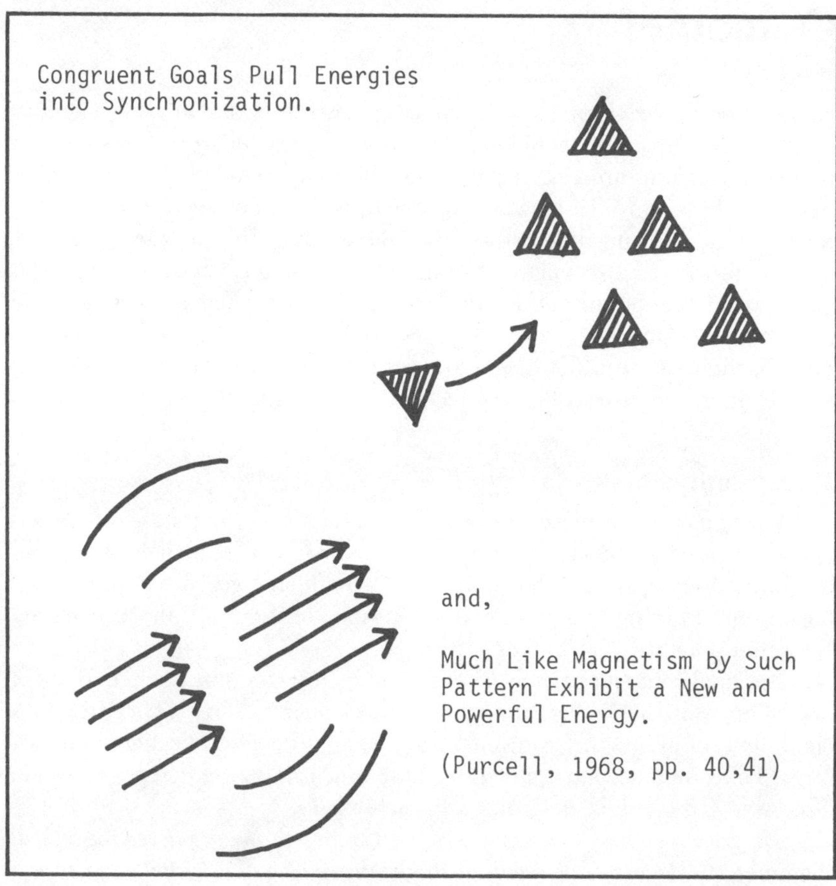
Congruent Goals Pull Energies
into Synchronization.
and,
Much Like Magnetism by Such
Pattern Exhibit a New and
Powerful Energy.
(Purcell, 1968, pp. 40,41)

network therapy, in which all members of the family organize to help one or more members, is another evidence of a single goal which pulls energies into harmony and thereby becomes more powerful.

However, the caution must be raised that the goal in itself must be clearly perceived. Negative goals have also been known to draw human energies to their service. The goal of synchronization of human energies in itself, rather than the pursuit of another, specific goal, is a seductive notion. However, once imposed, it can create a force against individuality.

Community Health Assessment

When was the last community celebration? What was celebrated? What is the community's usual pattern after resolving a conflict? Does the community put the extra energies to work efficiently toward the goal, or do these energies dissipate?

Outcomes

Health

Incongruent goals can be a force toward decay or toward growth. The force provided by the pain of conflicting goals within one system, one organism, can provide the goal of bringing incongruent goals into relationship. On the other hand, the force provided by conflicting goals within one system can serve as a repulsive force, driving different aspects of the system away from each other. The pressure provided by incongruent goals, when these goals remain unresolved, serves as a force toward entropy or disorder. The same force, when goals are brought into relationship, serves as a positive force, and negentropy (increased order) is the result. For the system to survive and to grow, the balance of forces must be in the positive, cohesive direction, or chaos and disintegration result.

Community Health

Incongruent goals in a community can also be a force toward decay or toward growth. Long-standing conflict of goals—perceived as irreconcilable—can pull the community apart. On the other hand, conflicting goals may provide the opportunity to bring groups with little previous relationship into contact and communication with each other.

A school conflict can draw parents from both sides of the tracks into honest discussion with each other, over the needs of their children. The need for a community health center can bring neighbors into communication with each other. Different perceptions about the same issue can draw different groups into discussion and eventual closer ties with each other.

The cohesive forces in community must outweigh the negative "sociofugal" (Sommer, 1974) *forces, or eventual randomness, lack of cohesion, and lack of integrity—in the sense of wholeness—*(Rogers, M., 1970) *will result.* In some communities, where one side of the tracks represents an entirely different community than the other side of the tracks, this is the obvious case. Perhaps some future issue can draw the two communities into relationship, perhaps it cannot.

Conflicting goals, on the other hand, may bring different groups within the community into relationship with each other, and thereby serve as a cohesive force in the end.

Community Health Assessment

What are the directions the forces resulting from conflicting goals appear to be taking? What is the community's traditional pattern? Do differing goals serve as forces of disintegration of relationships, or as forces for eventual cohesion?

Incongruent Goals Can Increase

the Force

Toward Entropy

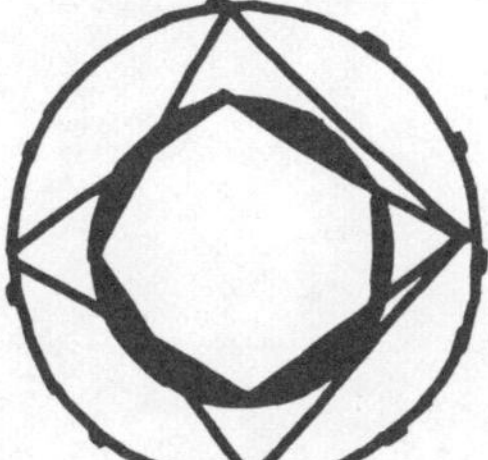

or,

by Means of the Intermediate
Step of Recognition, Provide
the Force to Bring Incongruent
Goals into Relationship.

References and Resources

REFERENCES

Arnstein, Sherry. A ladder of citizen participation. *Journal of the American Institute of Planners*, 1969, 35, 216–224.

Bennis, Warren, Benne, Kenneth, & Chin, Robert (Eds.). *The Planning of Change*. New York: Holt, Rinehart and Winston, 1969.

Chermayeff, Serge & Alexander, Christopher. *Community and Privacy*. Garden City: Anchor, 1965.

Eriksen, C. W. Perceptual Defense as a Function of Unacceptable Needs. *Journal of Abnormal and Social Psychology*, 1951, 46, 557–564.

Parmeggiani, P. L. Telencephalo-diencephalic aspects of sleep mechanisms. *Brain Research*, 1968, 7, 350–359.

Purcell, Edward. Parts and wholes in physics. In Walter Buckley (Ed.), *Modern Systems Research for the Behavioral Scientist: A Sourcebook*. Chicago: Aldine, 1968, pp. 39–44.

Rogers, Martha. *An Introduction to the Theoretical Basis of Nursing*. Philadelphia: F. A. Davis, 1970.

Sommer, Robert. Our airports are sociofugal, not sociopetal, and it's an outrage. *New York Times*, March 3, 1974, section 10, pp. 1, 14, 15.

Tart, Charles (Ed.). *Altered States of Consciousness: A Book of Readings*. New York: John Wiley, 1969.

RESOURCES

Aguilera, Donna, Messick, Janice, & Farrell, Marlene. *Crisis Intervention: Theory and Methodology*. St. Louis: C. V. Mosby, 1970.

Alinsky, Saul. *Reveille for Radicals*. New York: Vintage, 1969.

Argyris, Chris. Selections from the impact of budgets on people. In Joseph Litterer (Ed.), *Organizations: Structure and Behavior, Vol. 1*. New York: John Wiley, 1969, pp. 282–295.

Buckley, Walter (Ed.). *Modern Systems Research for the Behavioral Scientist: A Sourcebook*. Chicago: Aldine, 1968.

Clemence, Sr. Madeleine. Existentialism: a philosophy of committment. *American Journal of Nursing*, 1966, 66, 500–505.

Deikman, Arthur. Experimental meditation. In Charles Tart (Ed.), *Altered States of Consciousness. A Book of Readings*. New York: John Wiley, 1969, pp. 199–218.

Frankl, Viktor. *Man's Search for Meaning: An Introduction to Logotherapy*. New York: Washington Square, 1963.

Laing, R. D. *The Divided Self: An Existential Study in Sanity and Madness*. Harmondsworth, Middlesex, England: Penguin, 1960.

Litterer, Joseph (Ed.). *Organizations: Structure and Behavior.* (Second Edition.) Vol. I. New York: John Wiley, 1969.

Litterer, Joseph (Ed.). *Organizations: Systems, Control and Adaptation.* (Section Edition.) Vol. II. New York: John Wiley, 1969.

Milgram, Stanley. *Obedience to Authority: An Experimental View.* New York: Harper & Row, 1974.

Perrow, Charles. The analysis of goals in complex organizations. *Organizations: Systems, Control and Adaptation,* In Joseph Litterer (Ed.), Vol. II. New York: John Wiley, pp. 369–378.

Redfield, Robert. Levels of integration in biological and social systems. *Modern Systems Research for the Behavioral Scientist. A Sourcebook.* Chicago. Aldine, In Walter, Buckley (Ed), 1968, pp. 59–68.

Riesman, David. From "inner-directed" to "other-directed." In Amatai Etzioni & Eva Etzioni-Halevy (Eds.), *Social Change: Sources, Patterns and Consequences.* (Second Edition.) New York: Basic Books, 1973, pp. 410–420.

Rotter, Julian. Generalized expectancies for internal versus external control of reinforcement. *Psychological Monographs: General and Applied.* 1966, 80 (1). Whole No. 609.

Sheehy, Gail. *Passages: Predictable Crisis of Adult Life.* New York: Bantam, 1976.

Vickers, Geoffrey. The concept of stress in relation to the disorganizations of human behavior. In Walter Buckley (Ed.), *Modern Systems Research for the Behavioral Scientist. A Sourcebook.* Chicago: Aldine, 1968, pp. 354–358.

Wang, Virginia, Fonaroff, Arlene, & Dawson, John. Problem solving for common goals in two types of community agencies. *American Journal of Public Health,* 1975, 65, 809–817.

7

CHAPTER SEVEN

Relationship: Building Toward Synergy

Relationships are associations between various components of the system. They are "that which ties the system together" within itself, with similar systems, or with its suprasystem (Hall & Fagin, in Buckley, p. 82).

Relationships between people are the major sources of the highs and lows of life. They provide the joy of growing, discovering, sharing with others. They provide relief from loneliness, and satisfaction for the need to share experiences and feelings with other people.

In addition, relationships provide both stability and the stimulus for growth. Relationships are perhaps the basic underpinnings of the meaning of community for all of us.

> How can we, by our togetherness, create more beauty, more value, release more power? How can *our relationship* contribute effectively to a greater Whole—our community, mankind, or the Earth?
>
> How can it contribute health, growth, transforming energy to *that which our relationship realizes itself to be a part?* As a human body is a harmony of organic function, so our relationship should assume a function in the harmony of the great planetary organism, Man.(Rudhyar, 1972, pp. 150–151.)

Types

Health

Relationship is a basis ingredient of health. There are many types of relationships which can exist between or within human systems (people). I-Thou relationships carry all the warmth and energy of openness, sharing, caring, respect, and acceptance for each other (Buber, 1958; Maslow, 1971, pp. 155–199; Rogers, C. 1967). They are more characteristic of "horizontal" relationships within the community.

Me-It relationships depersonalize the other, are likely to be judgmental, and constitute a barrier to the conduction of the healing energies of caring, concern, openness, and respect for the other. They are characteristic of hierarchical, vertical, authoritarian relationships.

Both I-Thou and Me-It relationships can exist within an individual—between different parts of himself—those elements of self which he honors, values, and accepts or those parts of self which he rejects (Ehrich, 1969; Hjelle, 1969).

Community Health

Relationships are another one of the basic ingredients of both health and of community. Relationships provide the "meaning" of community—the communities of our past, present, and future—for all of us as individuals.

Both I-Thou and Me-It relationships can exist between members, members and groups, and groups within the community (Ryan, 1971; Shapiro, 1971; Suttles, 1968). The community's images of its young children, different ethnic groups, older people or warring gangs are likely to provide examples of different relationships between community groups.

I-Thou qualities of relationships are evidenced by the caretakers in both formal and informal channels in the community who take time to listen—the boundary workers in formal organizations who bend the rules to tailor services to individual needs, and the passers by who are willing to stop to help people on the street.

The board of a community agency may be able to make decisions on the basis of the needs of individuals or groups within the community (I-Thou) or be constrained to deal with cost effectiveness and program priorities as the basis of their decision making (Me-It). In reality, of course, in an age of scarcity, these elements overlap. Many individuals and groups are skilled at making I-Thou decisions simulate Me-It decisions for purposes of gaining program acceptance. The converse is also true.

Me-It or Us-Them relationships occur as a result of prejudice.and lack of knowledge and/or lack of acceptance between groups. Propaganda techniques designed to depersonalize the "enemy" during wartime, or the opposing group during union activities, are examples of attempts to create barriers to I-Thou relationships (Bennis, Benne & Chin, 1969, pp. 147–152).

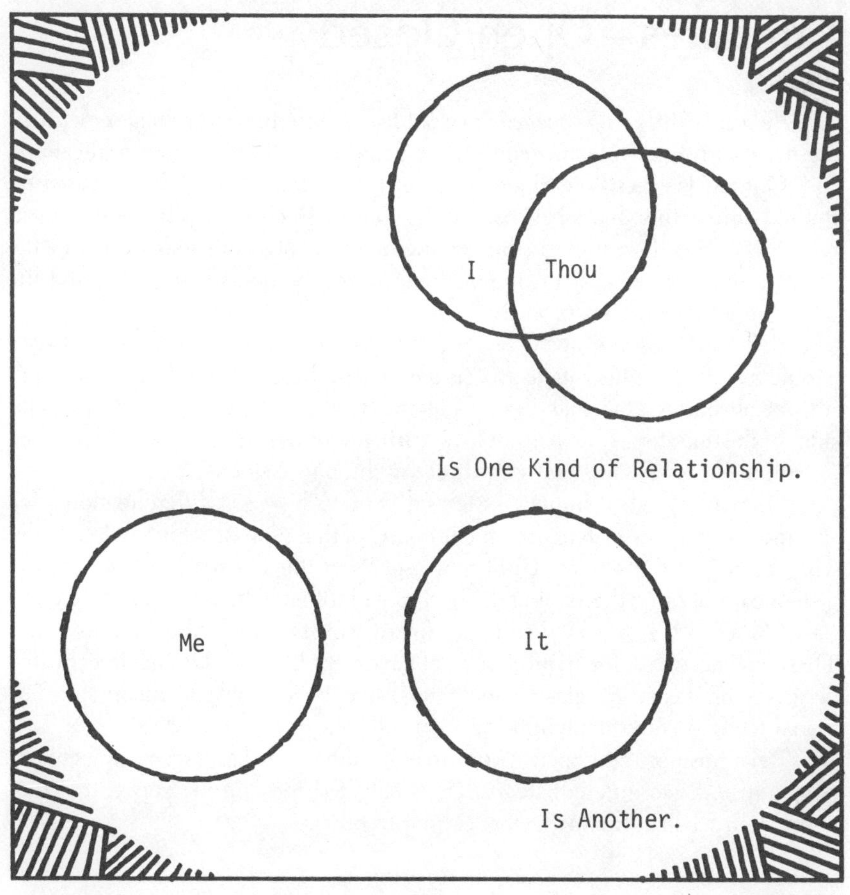

Relationships between the individuals and between the groups within the community are essential to the character, the well-being and the quality of life within the community.

Community Health Assessment

What indicators of I-Thou relationships can be seen in your community? What are the groups within the community that genuinely respect and care for each other? What indicators of Me-It relationships can be seen? What groups are prejudiced and misunderstand each other? How can you identify the relative proportion of each as environment for human interaction in your community? What ways can be seen to build I-Thou or decrease Me-It community relationships.

Attributes – Open/Closed

Health

Relationships can be opened or closed to communication to, from, or with all the parties involved. Health requires the presence of two-way communication.

Gordon Hearn's hotel-door model of human communication is based on the old connecting doors betweeen hotel rooms. Each side of the door had its own lock. Therefore the possibilities included having both doors open to the other, both doors locked, or one or the other of the doors being open and the other closed (Hearn, 1976, p. 29).

Relationships, and open, two-way communications are necessary between people in order to differentiate aspects of self, test these in the real world for their impact on others, and make value judgments about them. Openness on both sides of the door for expressions of love, caring for others, anger, self-esteem, and joy are all necessary for total growth of any human system.

Growth levels of human systems fluctuate between differentiation of a specific aspect of the system, and the bringing of that new aspect into relationship with the rest of the system. Until new aspects of the system are identified, the system cannot bring these into relationship with other elements of itself. (Gesell, Ilg & Ames, 1974, p. 27). The infant first discovers his mouth, then his hand. These are necessary for hand-mouth behavior to develop. The adolescent first discovers his sexuality, giggles and titters, and later is able to incorporate his sexual feelings comfortably into his own self-image.

Relationships, and open, two-way communications are necessary between people in order to differentiate aspects of self, test these in the very real world, and obtain feedback about their meaning to others.

Community Health

Relationships between sub-systems, or between individuals and the subsystems of a community may also be open, closed to each other, or some combination of the two.

One-way communications occur when an edict, or policy statement is given. They are most frequent in vertical relationships. The "Regs" of the U.S. Federal government (Federal Register) are regulations which spell out the ways in which a law is to be implemented. Attempts have been made to make them a two-way communication process. Once they have been published, a certain number of days are allowed for public response to their content before revisions are made, and they become final. Each step in this process is "one-way communication" and the large size of the systems involved make the process slow and nonspontaneous.

Two-way communications, as generallly known, occur in smaller, face-to-face groups, where rapid give and take, and discussion of the issues at hand may occur (Maternity Center Association, 1970).

No-Way communications (pun intended) occur when both sides are closed

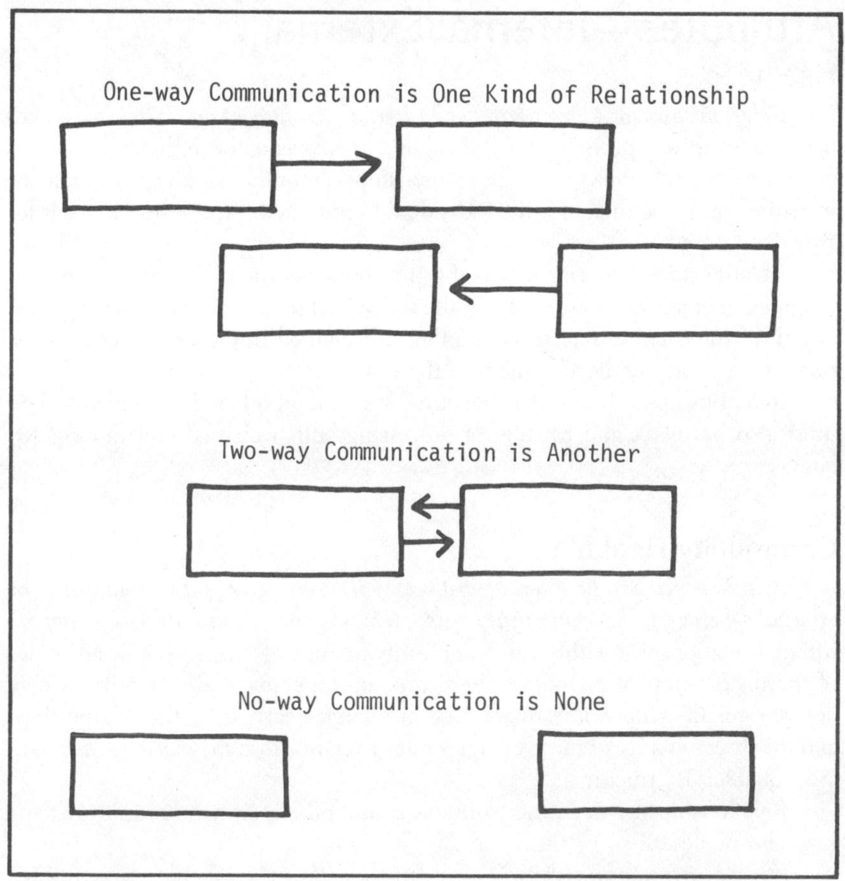

to communication with the other. They are an indicator of the presence of boundaries.

The matrix of values provided by the community affects the issues and areas of openness and closure for families, individuals, and friends, in school, at work, and in the recreational settings of the community.

The level of community openness to individuals and groups' mutual expressions of feelings and ideas reflects the level of development (or health) of the community itself.

Community Health Assessment

What are the areas of openness and closure of communication between groups within the community? What groups represent leading edges of openness to two-way communications within the community? What barriers to two-way communications exist?

Attributes – Internal/External

Health

Relationships may be internal or external to the system. They may exist between various aspects of the individual, or between the individual and his environment. Obvious, internal relationships—mouth, esophagus, stomach, intestine—must be intact for the individual to process the nutrients he needs for growth.

Relationships between less visible mechanisms for the processing of unweighted energies must also exist for the individual to grow. Intake, process, and output of information, caring, and other unweighted human energies must be intact for continuing development of the system.

Relationships between the individual system and others in its environment must also be intact and capable of processing both weighted and unweighted energies.

Community Health

Relationships can be internal, between various aspects of the community, or external—between the community and other systems within its environment. Internal relationships within the community include all the aspects or attributes of the distribution of energies. The degree of attraction and/or repulsion may describe relationships. The major type of energies carried by the relationships and the directionality of these energies in any relationship may also be described (See Chapter 3, "Energy").

Relationships between the community and other, extracommunity systems may also be described by means of the same attributes.

Internal relationships between the groups within the community would include, for example, the relationship between the Visiting Nurse Association and the hospital. The degree of openness or closure of the hospital to the requests for placement of a VNA coordinator within its walls, or the request of the hospital inservice department for the opportunity for its head nurses to make home visits with the VNA nurses, will be carried, by means of a relationship established in openness, understanding, and trust, or not, depending upon the history (quality of time) of their relationship.

External relationships between groups within the community and groups outside the community might include the relationship of the Visiting Nurses Association and the "Blues" or other third party payers. The relationship may be broad enough to allow consideration (two-way communication) of the need for payment for persons in the community with no acute medical diagnoses, but with many severe nursing diagnoses. This communication may be open from the VNA, closed on the side of the third party payers, or open on both sides. Once again, this depends on the history and trust established between the two groups and upon the ability to document the needs of the clients (the force with which the message enters the relationship's channels).

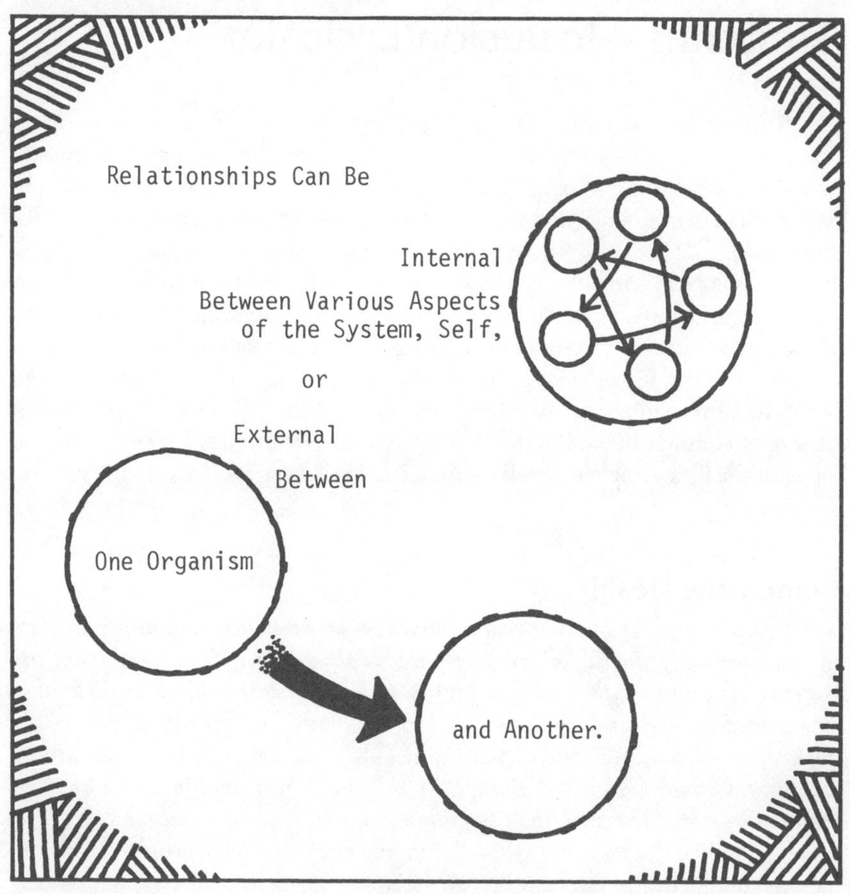

Relationships Can Be
Internal
Between Various Aspects
of the System, Self,
or
External
Between
One Organism
and Another.

Internal and external relationships must be intact and functioning for the community to pursue its growth. The development of new relationships must be able to occur as new needs and resources become available. The greater ease with which new relationships within the community and between the community and its suprasystem develop, the more rapid can be the community progress toward increasing health.

Community Health Assessment

Is there a pattern for the development of new relationships between different groups within the community? Is it one of long conflict and borderline resolution of issues, or is it one of little conflict and rapid progression toward a solution?

Attributes—Inclusion/Exclusion

Health

Relationships may include or exclude parts or wholes of self or other. Relationships, therefore, can be considered between parts of self, parts of self and parts of the environment, parts of self and the whole environment, whole self and parts of the environment, and whole self and whole environment (Hearn, 1976, pp. 27–29).

Physiological parts of self may or may not be in communication with each other, aspects of psyche may or may not be in relationship with each other (Luft, 1969, p. 13). Similarly, one's entire being may be in relationship with parts of the environment, as is the case with both positive energies, such as clear air and beautiful surroundings, or negative energies, such as chemical toxins. Health requires a continuing development of increasing relationships between different aspects of self, and between self and environment (Rogers, M., 1970, pp. 91, 97–101).

Community Health

Relationships within the community and between the community and its environment may include or exclude parts or wholes of self and environment. Different subgroups within the community may be in relationship with each other or excluded from relationship with each other. Those on the other side of the tracks may or may not attend P.T.A, health planning, or other community meetings. *Groups within the community may be in relationship with formal or informal groups external to the community.*

The public health nursing association may or may not be affiliated with the national public health association (American or Canadian Public Health Associations, for example). The local environmental group may or may not be affiliated with the Sierra Club or other environmental agencies. The nursing staff of the local agency may or may not belong to NCAP (National Coalition for Action in Politics). The local supermarket may or may not belong to a national chain.

Informal groups outside the community do exist on a national level, but are more difficult to identify. Interest groups and consequent networks of people sharing similar commitments do exist on an informal basis. These groups may be organized around interests varying from paper airplanes to human development and political action. However, they are not listed in the phone book, or in lists of formal agencies, and therefore are difficult to find until one plugs into the network, usually through an individual member.

The whole community is in relationship with aspects of its environment. All of the weighted and unweighted energies in the environment have their impact on the community as a whole. National economic forces affect employment and consequently the economic health of the community itself. Informational energies have their impact on the community by means of the values, goals, and perceived options for behavior and development in the community. Similarly,

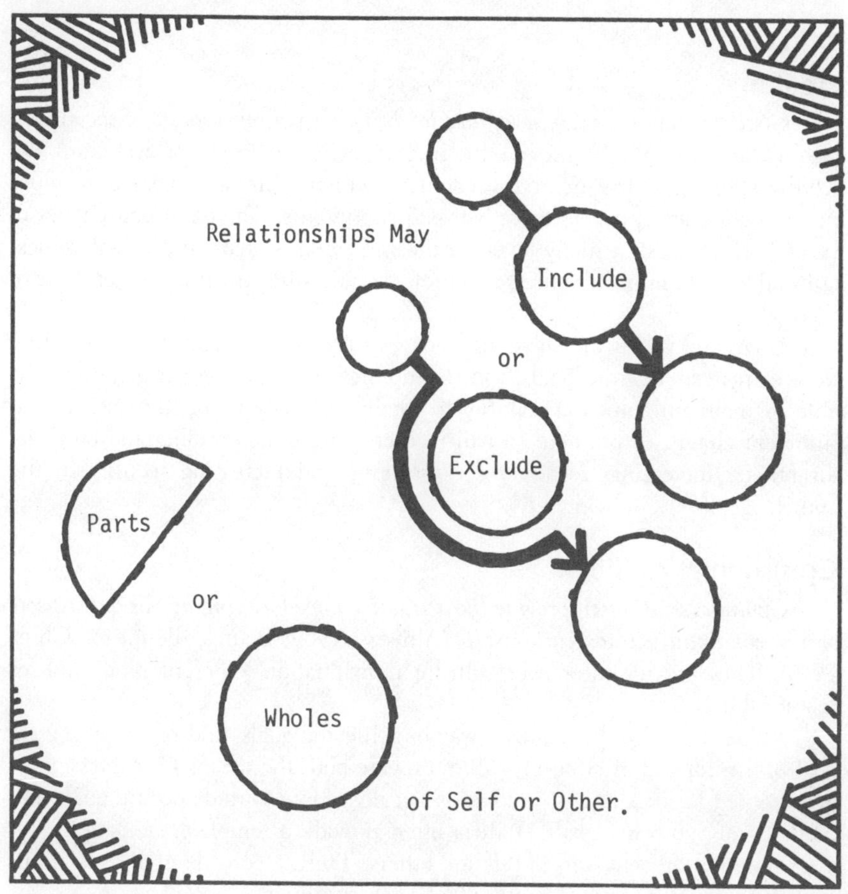
Relationships May
Include
or
Exclude
Parts
or
Wholes
of Self or Other.

sunspot activity affects many aspects of human life through its effects on weather, agriculture, and in other as yet unidentified ways.

Community Health Assessment

What aspects of the community are in relationship with each other? Which are excluded from relationship with other parts of the community? Which elements of the community are in relationship with which aspects of the environment? What are the formal groups and what informal groups related to the health needs of the community are in relationship with groups external to the community? What groups relevant to the community exist in the environment? Are the appropriate groups in the community in relationship with these?

Forces

Health

Goals provide the attractive force for bringing various aspects of the system into relationship. Values provide the individualized methods for evaluating the worth of goals, and the methods for achieving them. Similarly, goals and values may function as repulsive forces between subsystems. There are many types of values, which exist at many levels of the individual system. Individual values, cultural and community values, and professional values are examples of some of these.

Goals and values may be congruent, or they may be incongruent. In order for the organism to grow, goals, values, and methods for achieving goals must be able to maintain sufficient stability to retain the integrity of the system, and sufficient change to promote growth in increasing understanding and empathy for others, increasing freedom of expression, and increasing security in the knowledge of self (individuality).

Community Health

Common goals often provide the attractive force for bringing various aspects of the community into relationship (Alinsky, 1969; Bennis, Benne & Chin, 1969). They provide the power both for individuation (differentiation) and for relationship.

Values are an individualized way of achieving goals, and represent a great deal of the content of culture. Values provide both the means for expression of deep rooted feelings and a positive or negative force toward specific goals and methods of achieving goals. Values often provide a template, or pattern, for assessment of the behaviors of self and others. Trust, a core element of relationship, is rooted in perceived similarity of relevant values.

Values are communicated both overtly and covertly (Luft, 1969). Trust between community groups develops as the overt and covert messages remain congruent. Overt statements of values coupled with incongruent behaviors results in eventual mistrust between groups. The complexities of information networks in large bureaucracies are likely to produce incongruent behaviors, as people make statements, new information is obtained, and incongruent behaviors follow before information can be exchanged with all the groups affected by the decisions made.

Large amounts of information coming from various sources should affect the content and style of many decisions. Methods for coping with this amount of information need to be developed. Consistency of action and values is a basic human value required for trust, and consequently for developing and maintaining relationships. The steady bombardment of new information, conflicting information, and conflicting needs in a era of scarce resources makes it almost impossible for large organizations to maintain the appearance of consistent values and behaviors.

Incongruent goals and values can provide a significant stressor to individuals

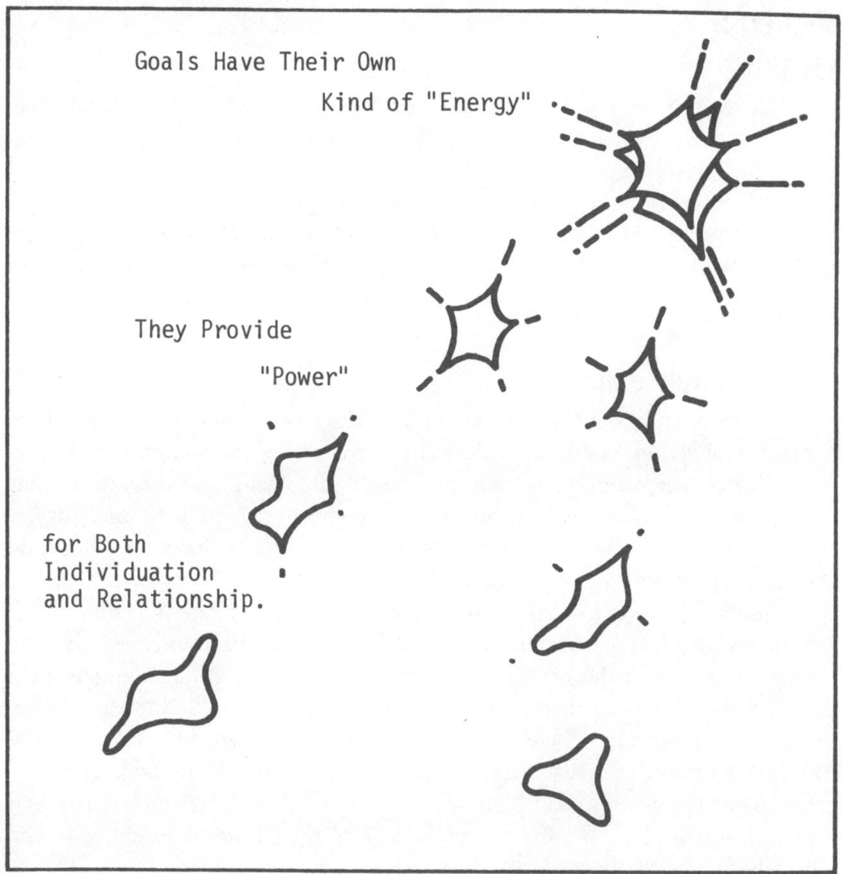
Goals Have Their Own
Kind of "Energy"
They Provide
"Power"
for Both
Individuation
and Relationship.

and groups within the community. Stressors, when they are perceived as controllable, and therefore resolvable, exert a positive force for health. On the other hand, stress, when the stressor is perceived as impossible to change, alter, or exert any influence upon, becomes a significant negative factor for health (Pellitier, 1977, pp. 5–6). Community stresses of both kinds may exist, and depend upon the interaction of the individuals and the causes of stress in the environment (Rogers, M., 1970, pp. 101–102).

Community Health Assessment

What are the areas of conflicting goals and values in the community? What are the most significant stressors to the individuals and groups within the community? Which groups perceive these as factors over which they can have some influence? Which groups see these as factors over which they are unable to exert any influences? What are the possible ways to assist them to perceive options for influence, and take active and successful steps to influence the stressors related to conflicting goals and values within the community?

VALUES

Health

Values are individualized ways of perceiving and achieving goals and function as "gatekeepers" in relationships. Trust and acceptance or rejection of aspects of self or others are rooted in large part in values.

Values exist on many levels and aspects of persons or community. Individual, cultural, and professional values can both close options and open directions for behaviors. Both individual and cultural values may be congruent or incongruent.

Community Health

Values of groups within the community also serve as gatekeepers, serving to open or close boundaries between different subsystems of the community. Values determining acceptance or rejection of prostitution within a community may close subgroups within the community to communication with each other, unless higher order values maintain communication and respect for others and thereby keep communications open.

Professional values on the priority of different types of care may differ. The hospital's obstetrical department may believe that hospitalization is necessary for the safe delivery of babies. The home birth group may feel that hospitals are a dehumanizing element in the birth experience. These conflicting values may prevent communication between these two groups. Overriding values might induce communication which could result in enrichment for both groups—greater safety for the home birth group by means of hospital back up services, and greater humanization for the hospital's clients by means of listening to the methods used by the home birth groups.

The use of native healers, shamans, or Christian Science practitioners may be discredited ("ruled out") by professionals, but held in high esteem by members of other groups within the community.

Nurses often serve as boundary workers in situations of conflicting cultural and professional values. The interpretation of the benefits of each approach to the members of the opposite group facilitates acceptance and consequently a broader range of perceived options.

Cultural conflicts exist on many levels. The members of transitional generations feel the conflict most acutely and internally. The teenage children of Puerto Rican families in New York are torn between the strict values of their parents and the liberal values of the urban American culture. The teenage children of some Middle European parents in North American feel the conflict between their parents' values on arranged marriages and North American values on marriages of choice. Generation gaps, culture shock, and change are all evidence of value stress—of conflicting values and inadequate time to resolve the conflicts which arise into new, acceptable, and broader options.

Value stress in formal caretaking organizations arises from formalized values

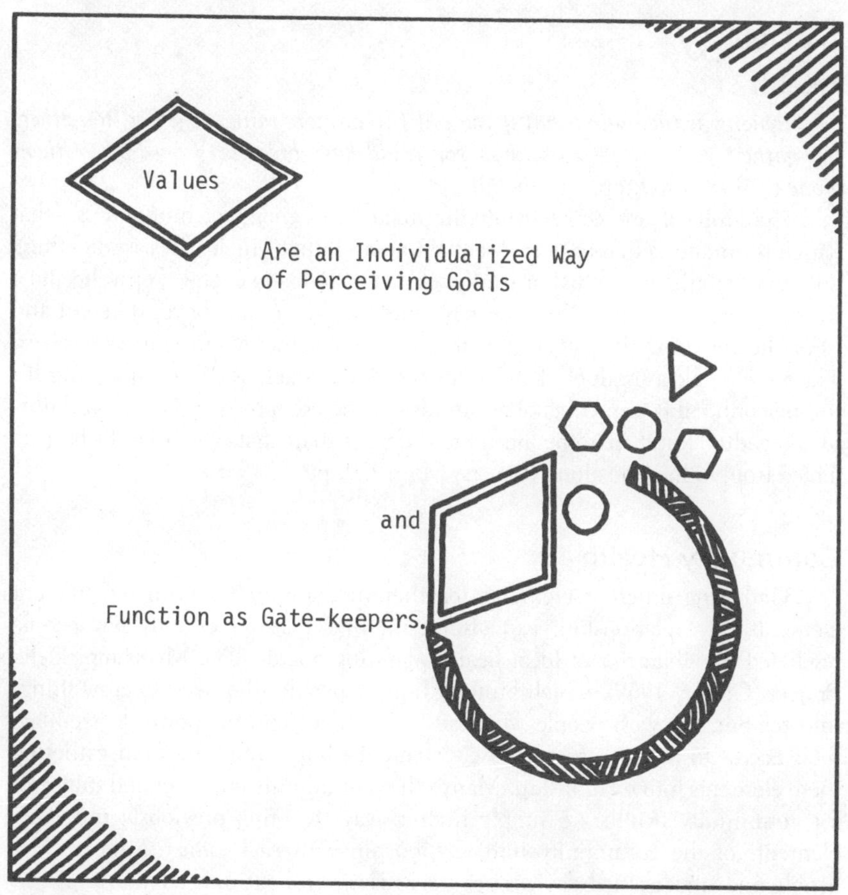

of high priority on the care of individuals and groups. This, coupled with the high need for survival in an era of scarcity, provides a significant stressor to the individuals within the organization, and to those groups it intends to serve.

Community Health Assessment

What values serve to prevent acceptance of each other by groups within the community? What values serve as internal stressors within groups within the community? What overriding values can be differentiated for use in building acceptance of the differentiating aspects of self or others?

Synergy

Health

Synergy is the notion that if you put two or more things together (to-gather, two-gather) you will get more than you could have predicted from both of them alone (Fuller, 1969, pp. 71, 76–99).

Certainly, if one can separate the matter and energy of humanness—that which is unique, different, and essential to man is that which arises as something different than the individual properties of matter added to energy. A psyche and a soma equal you, or me. We are each something over and above, different and unpredictable from the parts which are gathered together to form our own selves. The individual, a product of two different DNA codes, is still unique, and his full personhood is unpredictable from his genetic components. Nature and nurture together result in someone quite different than that which could be predicted from either one alone (Rogers, M., 1970, pp. 92–93).

Community Health

Gathering different elements together in community, bringing different elements into relationship, can also result in synergy. Certainly few people predicted the character of local health planning boards. The Mississippi Delta Project (Geiger, 1969), which brought hungry people who liked to grow things into relationship with people who had the concern and the power to facilitate their access to the soil, found a new element—hope, resulting from gathering these elements into relationship. Many other community programs and strategies for community health are simply finding ways to bring previously unrelated elements of the community into relationship with each other. Lonely older people and understaffed day care centers, when brought into relationship, can result in an increased richness of learning and feeling for both groups.

Something unique to the relationship emerges. It provides new energies and new capabilities as a result of its own unique quality.

We have much to learn about synergy in community, but one can often see its results when different groups in community begin talking to each other. New and creative solutions to problems arise, new perceptions of assets and options occur, and new abilities to get things done are often the result.

The women's movement, gathering interested individuals in the community together, did much to liberate men from the cultural restraints on their own personhood. Who could have predicted it? The ecumenical movement resulted in increased energy and creativity in its member churches.

Health care referral centers, by gathering information about all available sources of care, identify shortages in resources. They therefore gain information regarding the need to provide certain forms of care. Meals on Wheels programs bring the elderly-alone into relationship with the rest of the community, although often by a tenous thread. If this relationship is open to two-way communication (which takes time), those who provide the care must gain richness

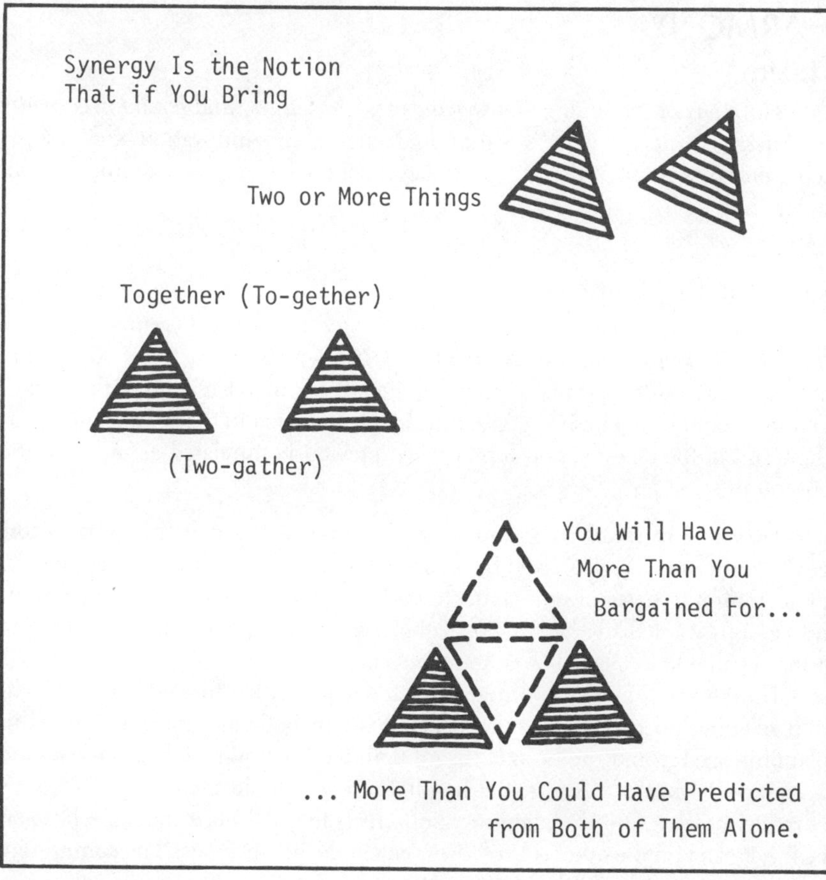
Synergy Is the Notion
That if You Bring
Two or More Things
Together (To-gether)
(Two-gather)
You Will Have
More Than You
Bargained For...
... More Than You Could Have Predicted
from Both of Them Alone.

from their contact with the older people. The caring that grows between nurses and their "clients" is over and above anything predictable, and perhaps a strong therapeutic force for both.

Community health requires the gathering together of individuals and groups that result in synergistic effects.

Community Health Assessment

Historically, which groups when brought into relationship, resulted in new and unpredicted behaviors? Who participated in establishing the Meals on Wheels program? Has anything unpredicted occured as a result? What groups participate in planning for community health? Has anything new and unpredictable occured as the result of bringing representatives of consumer groups into relationships with representatives of provider groups?

HARMONY

Health

Harmony of the timing and spacing of goals, values, and boundaries results in synergy. Synergy, with the increased energy and innovation that results, represents one phase of the activity-rest cycle of the developmental process in all living things.

Community Health

Harmony between groups within the community, when it occurs in terms of time, place, goals, and values, results in synergy. New energies, ideas, and activities can result in a burst of energies when these are released from the tasks of conflict resolution. These energies can then be directed to the tasks identified as the result of the new relationship between previously unrelated elements in the community.

Harmony of time. Harmony of time necessitates that the same needs, goals, and values are perceived by all at the same time. What good does it do if the community hospital now wants to build the hospital beds that the community groups wanted five years ago, if the community group now feels that the priorities should be placed on ambulatory care?

Harmony of place. Harmony of place requires that the elements brought into relationship can agree as to place. Perhaps both the community health planning agency and the hospital board both feel that 50 new hospital beds are necessary. Perhaps, however, the hospital wants to build them next door to its current facilities, and the planning group feels that the need for more hospital beds is greater on the other side of town, where no facility exists. The community groups want the hospital beds within their own neighborhood, so that they can visit and be visited more easily, if hospitalized. The hospital may feel that this is inefficient, and would result in lesser quality of care. No harmony of place can exist until some compromise can be achieved.

Harmony of goals. Harmony of goals occurs when newly related groups want to do the same thing. For example, The Children's Aid Society, the Department of Social Services, and the local women's liberation group may all want to establish a day care center. They may each differ as to their reasons for the goal, but they all agree to the same goal.

Harmony of values. Harmony of values occurs when all groups wish to do the same thing in the same way. For example, all the groups involved in wanting to build a day care center may agree that the focus should be on child development, rather than on a simple baby-sitting function. They agree that there should be supportive services for the parents to learn to understand and cope with their children more effectively. All groups agree that it is alright to give the children limited information about reproduction when the rabbits, guppies, or hamsters reproduce.

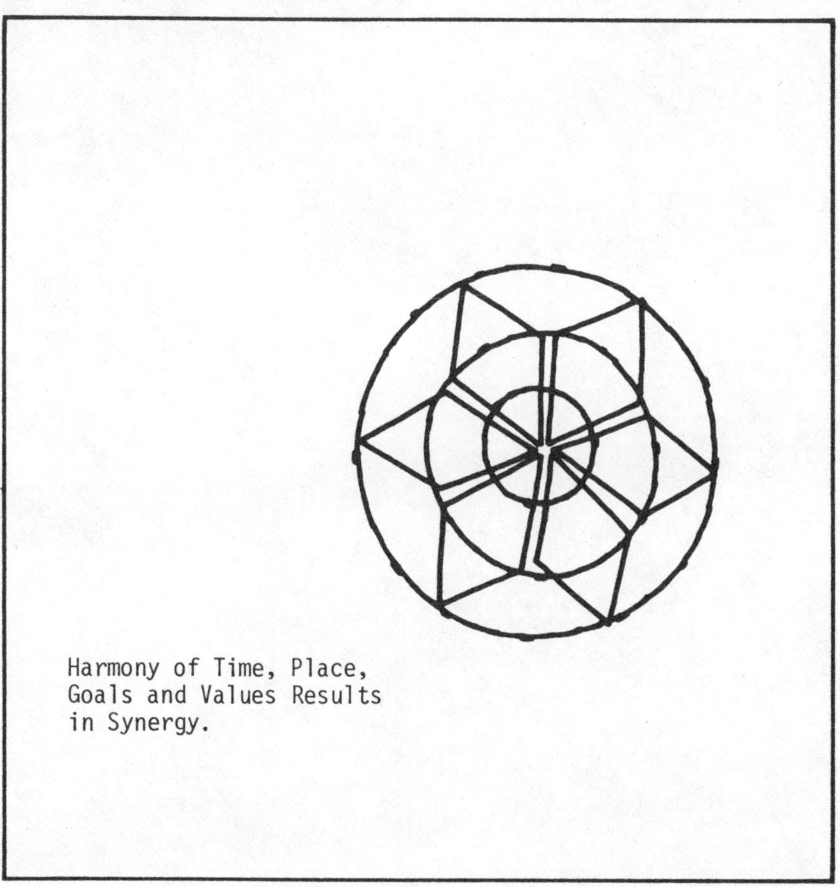

Harmony of Time, Place, Goals and Values Results in Synergy.

Synergy results when all these elements are in harmony. The more elements that can be brought into relationship, the greater the effects of the synergy that should be seen. However, full synergy in community rarely occurs, due to the number and complexity of elements in community. Synergy, when it is seen throughout a total community, is usually limited in time, and occurs in response to some disaster, survival threat, or dramatic occurance signalling a human need. Occasionally, a celebration will produce synergy within community.

Community Health Assessment

When was the last time that all the people in your community worked together toward a common goal? What was the happening or issue that brought them together? What developmental level did it represent—survival, safety, caring, or joy?

References and Resources

REFERENCES

Alinsky, Saul. *Reveille for Radicals.* New York: Vintage, 1969.

Bennis, Warren, Benne, Kenneth, & Chin, Robert (Eds.). *The Planning of Change.* New York: Holt, Rinehart & Winston, 1969.

Buber, Martin. *I and Thou.* (Second Edition.) New York: Charles Scribner, 1958.

Ehrlich, Howard & Lipsey, Carol. Affective style as a variable in person perception. *Journal of Personality,* 1969, 37, 522–540.

Fuller, R. Buckminster, Agel, Jerome, & Fiore, Quentin. *I Seem to Be a Verb.* New York: Bantam, 1970.

Fuller, R. Buckminster. Planetary planning. *The American Scholar,* 1971, *40,* 29–63, 285–304.

Geiger, H. Jack. The endlessly revolving door. *American Journal of Nursing,* 1969, 69, 2436–2445.

Gesell, Arnold, Ilg, Frances, & Ames, Louise. *Infant and Child in the Culture of Today.* (Revised Edition.) New York: Harper & Row, 1974.

Hall, A. D. & Fagen, R. E. Definition of system. In Walter Buckley (Ed.), *Modern Systems Research for the Behavioral Scientist: A Sourcebook.* Chicago: Aldine, 1968, pp. 81–92.

Hearn, Gordon. *The General Systems Approach: Contributions Toward an Holistic Conception of Social Work.* New York: Council on Social Work Education, 1969.

Hearn, Gordon. The client as the focal subsystem. In Harriet Werley, Ann Zuzich, Myron Zajkowski, & A. Dawn Zagornik (Eds.), *Health Research: The Systems Approach,* New York: Springer, 1976. pp. 25–35.

Hjelle, Larry. Personality characteristics associated with interpersonal perception accuracy. *Journal of Counseling Psychology,* 1969, *16,* 579–581.

Luft, Joseph. *Of Human Interaction.* Palo Alto, Calif.: National Press, 1969.

Maslow, Abraham. *The Farther Reaches of Human Nature,* New York: Viking, 1971, pp. 155–199.

Maternity Center Association. *A Dialogue Between Providers and Consumers of Maternity Care.* (Report of a One-Day Workshop held at and by Maternity Center Association on November 7, 1969). New York: Maternity Center Association, 1970.

Rogers, Carl. Learning to be free. In Carl Rogers & Barry Stevens *Person to Person: The Problem of Being Human: A New Trend in Psychology.* Lafayette, Calif.: Real People, 1967, pp. 47–66.

Rogers, Martha. *An Introduction to the Theoretical Basis of Nursing.* Philadelphia: F. A. Davis, 1970.

Rudyhar, Dane. Growth through relationship. *Fields Within Fields . . . Within Fields: The Metholodogy of Pattern*, 5, 149–152. New York: The World Council Institute, 1972.

Ryan, William. *Blaming the Victim*. New York: Vintage, 1971.

Shapiro, Joan. Group work with urban rejects in a slum hotel. In William Schwartz & Serapio Zalba (Eds.), *The Practice of Group Work*. New York: Columbia University, 1971, pp. 25–44.

Suttles, Gerald. *The Social Order of the Slum: Ethnicity and Territory in the Inner City*. Chicago: University of Chicago, 1970.

RESOURCES

Bennis, Warren, Berlew, David, Schein, Edgar, & Steele, Fred (Eds.). *Interpersonal Dynamics: Essays and Readings on Human Interaction*. (Third Edition.) Homewood, Ill.: Dorsey, 1973.

Giffin, Kim & Patton, Bobby (Eds.). *Basic Readings in Interpersonal Communication*. New York: Harper & Row, 1971.

Satir, Virginia. *Peoplemaking*. Palo Alto, Calif.: Science and Behavior, 1972.

Storm, Hyemeyohsts. *Seven Arrows*. New York: Harper & Row, 1972.

8

CHAPTER EIGHT

Pattern and Organization: Patterns and Process of Health

Pattern is the static description of structure. Organization describes the dynamic forces which move through, shape, reshape, and provide stresses on the existing pattern of community.

Pattern and organization, activity and rest, are seen in community health; the continuous process of differentiation, integration, and synergy in the community as a whole.

Overlapping Patterns

Health

Nodes, networks, and boundaries describe the mechanisms for storing, linking, and separating the energies in a living system. The pattern of the system as a whole must take into consideration the subpatterns for distribution of each form of energy and the relationships between each pattern as well.

Community Health

Overlapping patterns for the distribution of different forms of energy in the community will reveal a new, more complex pattern. Individual patterns for the distribution of individual energies are powerless to assist in the assessment of the health of the total community unless the relationship between the different patterns can be seen. This third dimensional look at the relationship between patterns provides the pattern for the community as a whole. It will reveal areas of congruence and incongruence, and nodes, networks, and boundaries of its own in a description of the system as a whole. Synergistic effects result from the relationships which exist. The relationship between political and healing networks may show a well-evolved set of linkages between both groups, or it may show linkages between only a few, partially representative members of the caretaking group and the political group.

Overlapping patterns between informational networks and political networks may show links and common channels between representatives of different political persuasions—or only a few—with some or all of the media.

Overlapping of the patterns for the distribution of caretaking and of informational energies may again show many highly developed and common channels and links—or few. Information about the political activities and stands of nurses may or may not be published in the media with the same force and frequency as that of physicians or hospital administrators.

The nodes, networks, and barriers of the patterns of interaction between healing, informational, and political energies, for example, provide a further description of the complexity of the community as a whole. The relationships between patterns for distribution of different forms of energy are rarely formalized. Most often they can be found only by methods aimed at identifying informal channels within the community. Only recently has lobbying—a formalized linkage between political and other forms of energy—won recognition in the helping professions. Information or public relations offices link nodes of industrial, healing, or other energies with the resources for carrying information.

One person often serves as node or link between two different patterns for energy distribution. These pivotal people, with overlapping spheres of influence, are important to identify in community, and often serve as resources for large amounts of information and influence. The boards of directors of nonprofit agencies often seek to obtain access to resources by means of selecting such individuals to their membership.

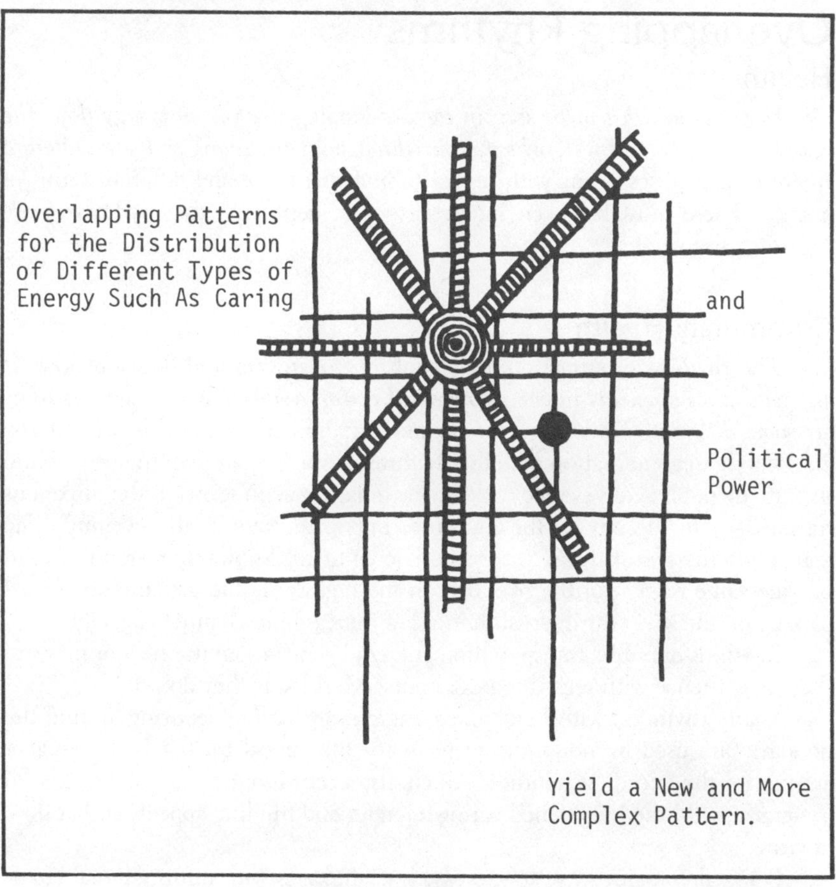

Overlapping Patterns
for the Distribution
of Different Types of
Energy Such As Caring
and
Political
Power
Yield a New and More
Complex Pattern.

Community Health Assessment

What is the pattern that emerges from looking at overlapping patterns for different forms of energy distribution in the community? What are the major links—what individuals or groups serve to bring different spheres of influence into relationship with each other?

Overlapping Rhythms

Health

Levels of health can be seen in the overlapping rhythms of energy flow, the pulses of activity and rest, which occur throughout the living system. Different rhythms and pulses occur with regard to both the same and different forms of energy. These must be taken into account in identifying the rhythms of the organism as a whole.

Community Health

The rhythms of attraction and repulsion, of inward and outward flows *of different forms of energy in community will reveal overlapping pulses–some similar some different.* Daily rhythms of transportation of people into the city by automobile in combination with the rhythms of transportation of the people into the city by public conveyance will show similar times in terms of the directions travelled—into the city in the morning, out of the city in the evening. The congestion that results from this is well known to all. Subways or monorails can provide some respite for the overload on the highways, and prohibition against parking on the street during rush hours can increase the channel capacity.

Rhythms of public transportation and emergency room use may or may not show congruence with regard to peak hours. Most likely they do not.

Yearly rhythms, with heightened energies for caring occuring around the holidays, are used by nonprofit agencies for the appeal for funds. Newspaper appeals for the "neediest families" which also occur around the holidays add to (synergize with) the heightened caring energies and funding appeals at that time of year.

Political energies strive to increase their linkages with informational channels around election times, and the media both increase their input and output of political information during election times. Other groups strive to build new links with political candidates. Candidates strive to increase their communication with their constituents and with special interest groups.

Horizontal and vertical directions of energy flow within the community as a whole provide other indicators of the health of the community. Formal decision making may follow a vertical, top down (authoritarian), or bottom up (democratic) model. In either case, one group serves the will of the other. On the other hand, information may be communicated equally from the top down and from the bottom up. Joint decision making may therefore be carried out with all members of the group contributing equal amounts from different, but equal, vantage points.

Informal caring energies may be carried horizontally, and formal healing energies carried vertically. Economic energies used to support formal healing energies may be imported from sources outside the community—state or Federal funds for example, or be gathered from within the community itself (United Way appeals for example).

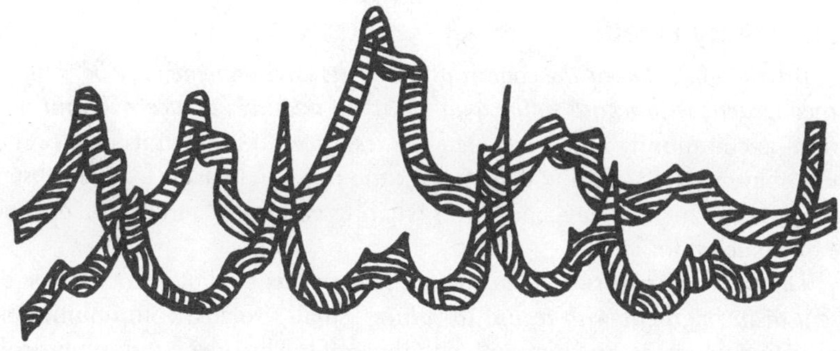
Overlapping Rhythms of Energy Flow,
The Pulses of Activity, and Rest, also Occur in Community.

The direction and force of energy flowing within the community are shaped by the goals of groups within the community and of the community as a whole. In addition, the rhythms of energy flow within the community create stresses on community patterns for the distribution of energy. These stresses may include the need to carry more of the relevant resources, to carry additional resources, to carry the resources to new and different aspects of the community, or to gather resources from more elements of the community. Such stresses result from and produce further pressure to redefine community goals, thereby providing the forces for continuing development of the community.

Community Health Assessment

What overlapping rhythms, point and counterpoint of the community's rhythms, create stress in the community? What additional resources need to be carried? What groups require the resources? What additional resources need to be gathered from within the community?

Community and Environment

Health

Identification of the interactions between the system and its environment reveal additional stresses and strains, resources and needs, that arise from this interaction. Congruent and incongruent resources and needs, congruent and incongruent goals and values, congruent and incongruent rhythms of energy flow may result in either stress or synergy in the interaction between the community and its environment.

Community Health

Interaction between the community and its environment may be congruent or incongruent with regard to the availability of resources to meet relevant needs. A mining community may have adequate resources to mine in its environment. These may, in time become depleted, or the outside demand for the substance may slacken—such as happened with whaling communities and the decreased use of whale oil for lamps.

The interaction between the community and its environment may be congruent or incongruent with regard to values. Small, isolated communities often have values which are incongruent with those of the broader community around them. This occurs in some religious communities, which do not accept medical interventions. Incongruent values may also occur in small, deviant communities, such as communities of alcoholic men, who do not place the same relative value on shelter as middle class groups.

The interaction between community and its environment may be congruent or incongruent with regard to rhythms of energy flow. The community may need to take in a relevant resource at a rhythm that fits or does not fit its availability in the surrounding environment. Communities in politically oppressed countries may feel the need for increased information about political happenings just as censorship increases.

Areas of incongruence of resources, needs, values, and rhythms of energy flow between the community and its environment create stresses and strains within the community.

Areas of congruence of resources, needs, goals, values, and rhythms of energy flow may create synergistic effects between the community and its environment.

A community's need to redefine its health planning mechanism may be synchronized with new national legislation producing the goals, values, economic, and information resources to pursue such a need. In such a case, the community's need for information is backed up by large amounts of information about health planning in the journals, in the media, and in specially produced publications. Further interest is stirred in members of the community who are drawn to the effort, and additional internal resources are built by the external resources. Financial assistance for planning mechanisms, salaries, space, telephones, and postage are provided by state and local funds. These resources provide further synergistic effects in aiding the task of network building in the

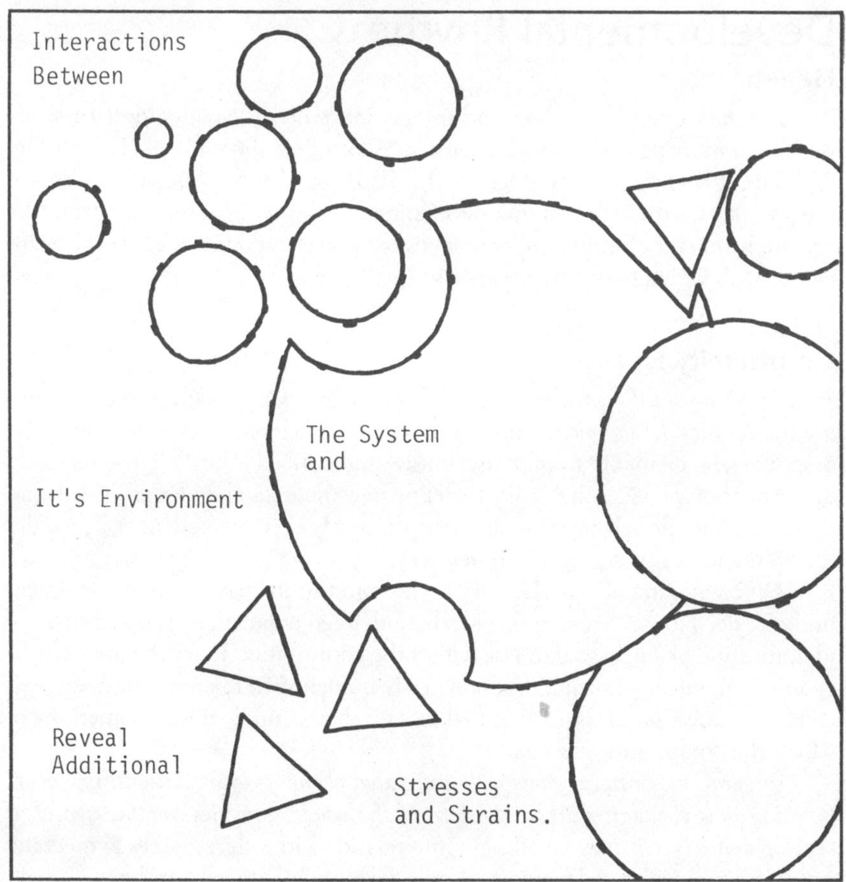
Interactions
Between
The System
and
It's Environment
Reveal
Additional
Stresses
and Strains.

local community. They also bring still more elements of community into relationship with a defined task.

On the other hand, incongruent needs may be seen between the community and its environmental forces. A community may have defined its priority of need as that of developing recreational resources at the time when national priorities have identified medical care as the overriding goal. Tax resources and human interest are drawn to these other tasks, rather than those internally defined by the community itself.

Community Health Assessment

What are the areas of congruence and incongruence between the community's needs and the resources available in the environment? What are the areas of congruence or incongruence between the community's values and those prevalent in its environment? What are the areas of congruence or incongruence with regard to the community's rhythms and those of its environment?

Developmental Rhythms

Health

Rhythms of differentiation and integration provide the basic pattern of development in living systems (Chermayeff & Alexander, 1965, p. 142; Gessell, Ilg, & Ames, 1974, pp. 22–26; Rogers, M., 1970, pp. 61–65. Stresses and strains provide the need for continuing development. The synergy resulting from the accomplishments of each developmental step provide additional energy and efficiency with which to pursue new goals.

Community Health

Rhythms of differentiation and integration provide the pattern for continuing community development. Stresses produce the need to differentiate, identify, describe new elements from a previously undescribed whole. The process of differentiation provides the ability to define new methods and new goals. Integration, building the relationship between previously described elements, provides the ability to pursue new goals in new ways.

Differentiation of new elements in the community may consist of identification of a need for service in a previously undefined population. It may consist of identification of a new goal or task within the community. It may be the identification of an already existing, but previously unidentified resource. In essence, it is the identification of something that previously was unidentified, something of which the community was unaware.

Integration, bringing previously unrelated elements into relationship, incorporating new elements into the pattern of the whole, provides another aspect of development. Needs may be brought into relationship with resources to meet the needs. Groups with overlapping goals may be brought into relationship with each other so that they may work together toward similar goals. Preexisting networks to carry one kind of resources may be brought into relationship with nodes to provide supplementary resources. New elements in community must be differentiated if new relationships are to be built.

Community Health Assessment

The essential task of community health assessment is to perceive the community's resources and needs accurately in order that strategies can be developed which are congruent with the community's developmental needs. Respect for the timing and rhythms of differentiation and integration is necessary if strategies are to be effective. A community's need to identify (differentiate) its own next developmental task may be the critical need, or the community may well be aware of needs, but require assistance to identify resources to meet the needs, or to build links between identified resources and needs.

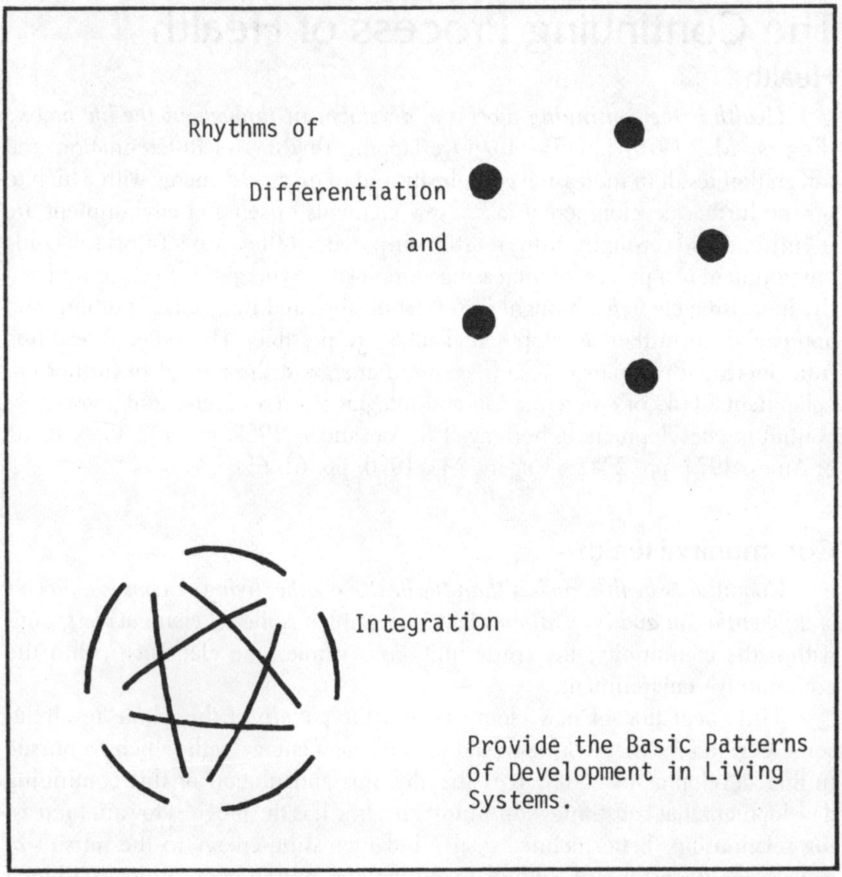

Rhythms of

Differentiation

and

Integration

Provide the Basic Patterns of Development in Living Systems.

The Continuing Process of Health

Health

Health is the continuing process of development throughout the life process (Rogers, M., 1970, pp. 55–60). Overlapping rhythms of differentiation and integration result in increasing complexity and in increased energy with which to pursue further developmental taks. New elements of self-and-environment are identified and brought into relationship with other aspects of self-and-environment in a process of increasing complexity. Synergistic effects result from the increasing elements brought into relationship, and innovative solutions and approaches to further developmental tasks are possible. The synergy resulting from increased complexity also frees more energy to the pursuit of further developmental tasks of differentiation and integration in a never-ending process of continuing development (Chermayeff & Alexander, 1965, pp. 142; Gessell, Ilg & Ames, 1974, pp. 22–26; Rogers, M., 1970, pp. 61–65).

Community Health

Community health, no less than the health of other living systems is a process of differentiation and integration of an increasing number of elements or groups within the community, the community as a whole, and elements within the community's environment.

The integration of new elements into the pattern of the whole results in some degree of synergy, a new pattern, and new energy with which to pursue further developmental tasks. It is the rhythms and motion of this continuing development that constitutes community health. It is the progress toward increasing relationship, better defined goals, and increasing energy to the pursuit of goals, which constitutes health in living systems, and in community as a living system.

Community Health Assessment

Community is a major environmental force for the health of individuals and families. Accurate assessment of levels of community health and the consequent development of appropriate strategies for community health can do much to facilitate wellness of the individuals and families who reside within the community.

Conclusion

The concepts which have been presented in this book are meant to be taken and used in whatever community you have selected as your system. Different concepts and their relationships will be appropriate depending upon the WHAT and WHY of your community and the reasons for assessing it. Testing these

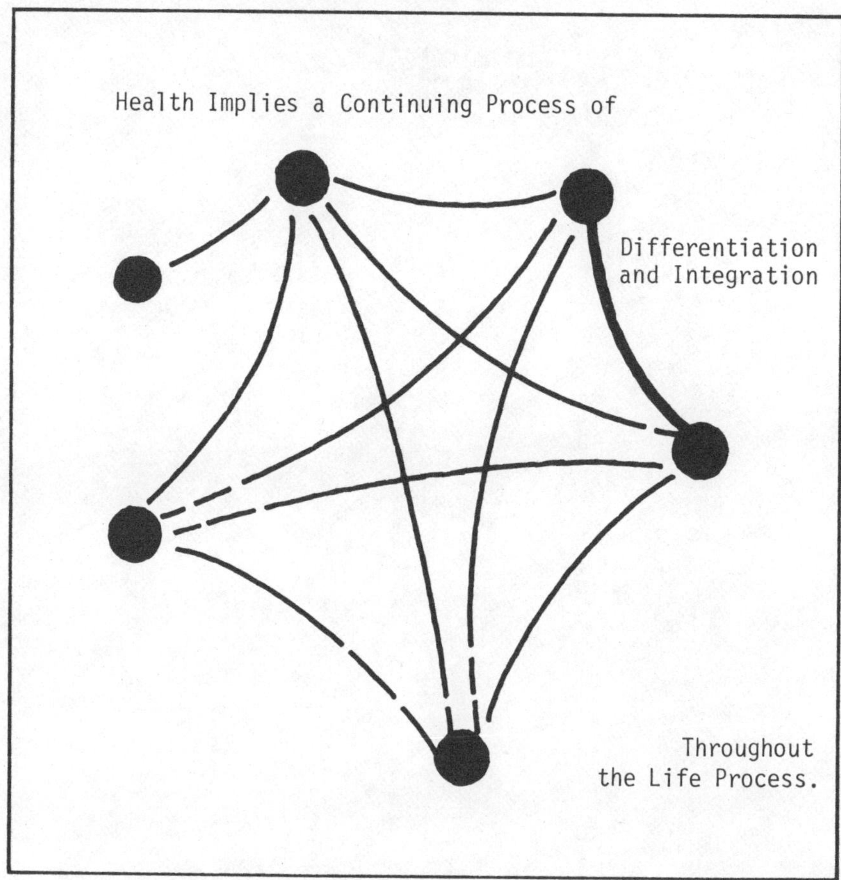
Health Implies a Continuing Process of
Differentiation
and Integration
Throughout
the Life Process.

concepts in the reality of individual communities, identifying the new concepts which result from such use, and building the relationships between them will result in new concepts, new relationships, and, therefore, new knowledge and approaches to the process of community health assessment.

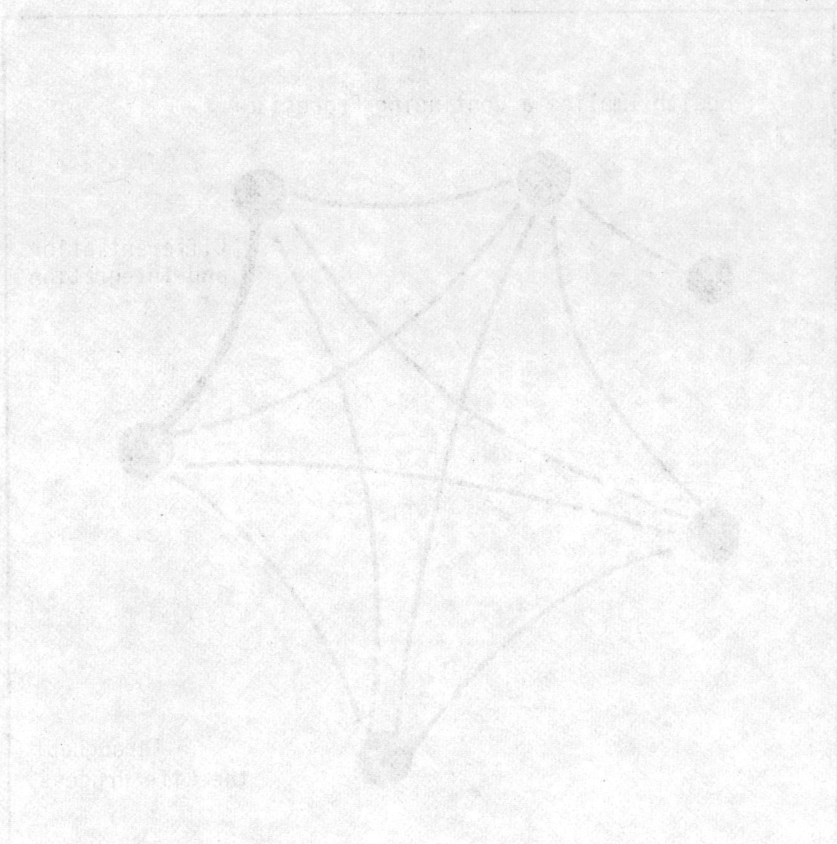

References and Resources

REFERENCES

Chermayeff, Serge & Alexander, Christopher. *Community and Privacy*. Garden City: Anchor, 1965.

Gesell, Arnold, Ilg, Frances, & Ames, Louise. *Infant and Child in the Culture of Today*. (Revised Edition.) New York: Harper & Row, 1974.

Rogers, Martha. *An Introduction to the Theoretical Basis of Nursing*. Philadelphia: F. A. Davis, 1970.

RESOURCES

Bennis, Warren, Benne, Kenneth, & Chin, Robert (Eds.). *The Planning of Change*. New York: Holt, Rinehart and Winston, 1969.

Gibb, Jack. *Trust: A New View of Personal and Organizational Development*. Los Angeles: The Guild Tutors Press, 1978.

Halprin, Lawrence. *The RSVP Cycles: Creative Processes in the Human Environment*. New York: George Braziller, 1969.

Fuller, R. Buckminster. Planetary planning. *The American Scholar*, 1971, 40, 29–63, 285–304.

INDEX

Pages in italics refer to pages where the definition appears.

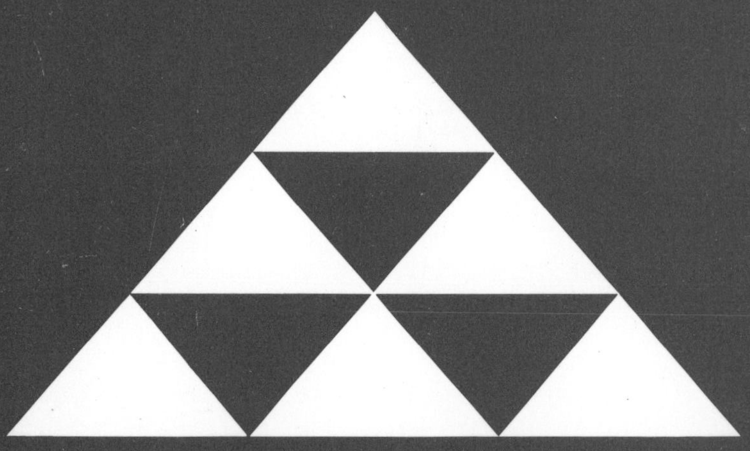

The first book on assessment of the community as a system!

Through a nursing perspective, this practical guide highlights:

▲ the concept of *community* as the focus for nursing assessment and intervention, to show how community forces affect the health of individuals and their families

▲ a *general systems* approach, with realistic applications

▲ unique tools for increasing community health assessment skills, emphasizing quality rather than quantity of care

▲ conceptual illustrations to enhance your understanding of the material

WILEY MEDICAL

JOHN WILEY & SONS

605 Third Avenue

New York, N.Y. 10016

New York • Chichester • Brisbane • Toronto

ISBN 0-471-34776-0